Performance and Sports Nutrition

Handbook with nutritional factors that can influence physical performance

Cristina & Olivier Rebière

Cristina Botezatu

ISBN-13: 9781790649785

TABLE OF CONTENTS

Introduction

We welcome you on your first guide within the new collection "SportPRO: Performance and Sports Nutrition" which we hope will help you learn to better control the factors that affect athletic performance.

This guide is made for all athletes, but especially sports enthusiasts who seek to reach performance and for those who are already elite athletes as well, who want to better understand mechanisms and effective levers they can use to increase their capacity. This book was voluntarily written in an accessible language, even if it is aimed at sport performance. Its purpose is to familiarize you with several concepts that have a big impact on your results. This is the first of a series that we want to develop and in which we will gradually discuss of increasingly sophisticated topics that will allow you to access or maintain a high level of performance.

Cristina Botezatu will share with you its research data, practical experiences and results and the methods applied in optimizing the performance of athletes who managed to climb the highest step of the Olympic podium. She has coached several athletes preparing for Olympic Games and World Championships in various sports: athletics, tennis, fencing, swimming, volleyball, handball, football, etc. Each sport has its own specificities and acts on biological, neurological and psychological specific mechanisms. We will help you know them better and learn to master them in order to fully optimize your athletic performance.

We invite you to start right away!

Sports performance and its mechanisms

Athletic performance is the combination of a complex training that is influenced by many factors that must be not only known, but considered and optimized during training to maximize the performance of the athlete.

The exceptional value of sports performance requires continuous improvement in all aspects of the preparation of athletes, the environmental conditions of their training, and their coaching as well. Whatever the practiced discipline and the level of performance achieved, sport performance is driven through continuous preparation at all levels without neglecting any aspect because, it needs a balanced workout that takes into account all the morphological mechanisms of the body. The expected high value of achievement, combined with the possibility of future growth, depends directly on the effort and the accuracy of the training conducted by the athlete and the seriousness of the approach towards many factors determined in sports training including psychological, biological, social aspects.

Vladimir Nikolaevic Platonov, a Russian scientist in the field said that: *"Performance is the expression of maximum individual possibilities in a field at some point."*

Indeed, there are several factors to specifically define and optimize in order to achieve athletic performance.

Let's find them out within the following sections:

Endurance

Endurance plays a very important role in most sports because it consists in the ability of an athlete to maintain an effort for a prolonged period, exceeding its limits, despite the fatigue.

Endurance requires great adaptability, involving the development of phenomena that may balance biological processes throughout the efforts to reduce energy consumption.

Increased resistance is conditioned by several factors that can influence more or less its manifestation:

☞ Maximum oxygen consumption or maximum volume of oxygen (VO_2max), because resistance is based on glycogen energy, fatty acids and lipids decomposition in the presence of oxygen.

☞ Type of muscle fibers

☞ Quantity and quality of energy resources, enzyme activity and hormonal regulation mechanisms

☞ Cardiovascular system capacity, breathing, muscle and other body functions to support the effort

☞ Level of development of motivational qualities (perseverance, determination, bravery)
☞ Level at which the central nervous system performs the coordination of the locomotor system and vegetative functions
☞ Age and sex

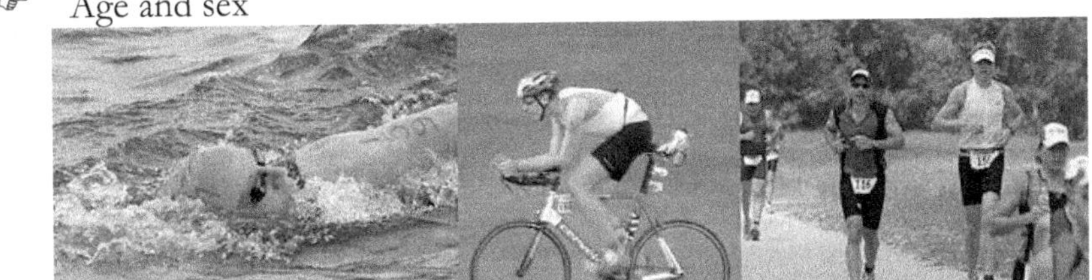

During resistance training, the functional activity of the body runs a series of changes that contribute to energy production in both aerobic and anaerobic conditions. The spent efforts during resistance tests is primarily of aerobic origin. These efforts are characterized as low intensity, medium or submaximal and are carried out under conditions of a balance between demand of, and oxygen supply. They can be kept for a period of several minutes to several hours depending on the intensity with which they occur. Aerobic power is limited by the capacity of the cardiorespiratory system to transport oxygen in the body. Improving the transport capacity of the O_2 to the muscle fiber is a priority of the resistance training process. In such cases, the long-term training in aerobic regime alternates with various intensities activities. Thus, the body recovers and can therefore increase the durability of the aerobic power.

During resistance training, a number of adaptations of the cardiovascular system are made within the body of the athlete. These adjustments are accompanied by an increase in heart volume, expansion of the heart chamber along with the growth of residual volume. The increased stroke volume occurs simultaneously with the rise of the heartbeat intensity, which promotes the emptying of the heart chamber. The improvement of microcirculation due to proliferation and use of the capillary network within skeletal muscles increases the contact ability between blood and muscle tissue, developing the ability to supply the muscle with power and oxygen.

Motivation is a key factor in resistance training because when fatigue sets in, the athlete can maintain the intensity level if it is supported by his will, which commands the nerve centers to continue - or even intensify - the effort, especially at the end of the race.

There are several types of endurance, particularly in relation to the period during which it must play its part:

🕐 Short term: endurance concentrated between 45 seconds and 2 minutes ; the amount of energy required is produced primarily by the anaerobic system.

🕐 Medium term: this endurance manifests from 2 to 8 minutes, when the aerobic sector gets more involved in the production of the required energy.

🕐 Long term: this is the stamina to longer efforts, more than 8 minutes, and for which energy production is mainly provided by the aerobic system.

Latest discoveries in the field of physiology and biochemistry have shown that the physiological mechanism of resistance is located deep within the muscle cells. This indicates that the primary training requires specific changes at the cellular level in skeletal muscles. That phenomena cause changes in blood flow within the cardiovascular circulatory system and other systems. A specific resistance level of development is due to the use of oxygen, appropriate and balanced at all levels (absorption-use-disposal) in order to not limit the functionality of the entire system.

Strength

Strength is the ability to overcome or withstand external resistance through muscular tension. These are created by a slide mechanism of actin filaments between those made of myosin. Actin and myosin are the two proteins by which energy is produced. This mechanism is actually the result of the formation of "union bridges" between myosin heads and some actin filaments. Through a chemical reaction, energy is released thereby generating a force directly proportional to the number of actin-myosin bridges formed. On this occasion, the inner muscle chemical energy is converted into mechanical energy.

This force is proportional to the number of muscle fibers which are recruited, and it greatly depends on the workout. The more fibers that come into play and the strength will be greater. The frequency of nerve impulses also affects the level of force. During low intensity exercises, the recruitment of fibers is done haphazardly, but when the intensity increases, recruitment becomes more organized, tending to sync up and having, as a result, intramuscular coordination.

In conclusion, the level of force depends on how the motor unit (UM) is involved.

The factors that determine the manifestation of the force are:

☑ The diameter of the muscle fiber

☑ The frequency of the pulses transmitted by the motor neurons to muscles

☑ The types of muscle fibers

☑ The amount of energy in the muscles

☑ The muscle fiber contraction rate

☑ The quality and integrity of the supporting bodies

☑ The recruitment of motor units

☑ Psychological factors

☑ Age and sex, etc.

With the extended training process, an increase in muscle mass is obtained, which may be due either to the thickening of the muscle fibers either to the proliferation of muscle fibers. Muscle fibers can be either type 1 or type 2, this characteristic being given by the myofibrils.

The muscle fiber type 1, known in the specialized literature as "slow-twitch" or "red fibers" are resistant to fatigue and are characterized by a slow contraction of the rich reserves of glycogen, enzymes of aerobic metabolism, a mitochondria lot relative to the sarcoplasm, a high catabolism, a high capillary density, neuron innervation alpha engines with a relatively low speed sending continuous nerve impulses sequences, characterizing sustained motor activity (e.g. the maintenance of posture).

Two types of fast fibers called "white fiber" are not resistant to fatigue. They are characterized by a rapid contraction of rich ATP reserves type phosphate compounds (adenosine triphosphate) and CP (phosphocreatine), a high concentration of enzymes required to anaerobic metabolism, a larger diameter than that of the type 1 fibers. innervation is performed by alpha

motor neurons at high speed, that transmit nerve impulses staple typical of voluntary motor activities of high intensity and short duration.

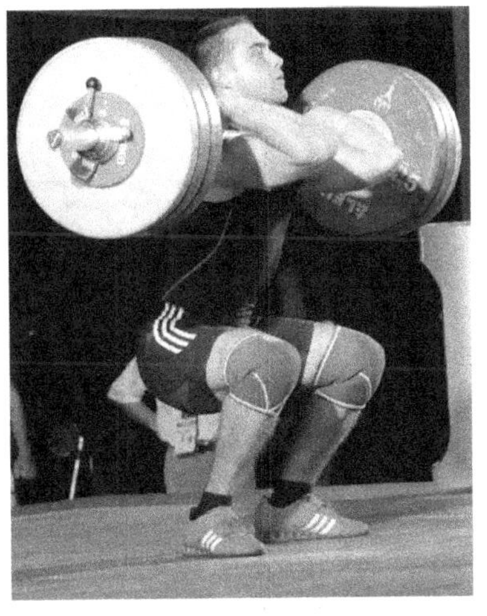

Inside a muscle, there are two types of muscle fibers, but certain muscles are mostly faster and others slower, depending on the number of predominant fibers.

The amount of energy possessed by the muscle fibers depends largely on the power of the athlete. A proper diet provides a lot of energy (ATP, PC, glycogen) and enzymes in the muscle fibers, blood and liver, allowing full effort deployment.

The quality and integrity of the support bodies are represented by the development of ligaments, tendons and bones.

The maximum muscle contraction begins first as the result of the slow motor units' contraction, ending with the contraction of the fast units. The recruitment of motor units and the frequency increasing of nerve impulses contribute to the increase in strength between 0 and 80% of the maximum possibilities. They represent the basic factors for the development of maximum strength.

There are several schemes of muscle contraction:

☞ The static or isometric diet when muscle length does not change. For example, the cladding exercises are done under the isometric contraction regime.

☞ The concentric dynamic regime: the muscle contracts by bringing its insertion points on the bones.

☞ The plyometric regime: the muscle contracts, initially eccentrically then shortens and works concentrically. This type of training helps to multiply the capacity to produce a more powerful movement within a very short period.

☞ Eccentric dynamic regime, during muscle lengthening, thanks to the insertions moving away.

As the force is considered the "foundation" of other factors influencing sports performance, it should not be neglected, regardless of the practiced sport. It requires well-defined compliance in order to be effective and not to cause any injury.

Here are the requirements:

1. Know the level of force and the athlete's physical capacities
2. Choose wisely the exercises for the development of force depending on the specific sport.
3. Accurately determine the workload
4. Determine the intensity depending on the capabilities of the athlete
5. Provide individualized recovery break adapted to each athlete
6. Develop a force preparation plan

Speed

Speed is equal to the ratio between the distance and time taken to travel a given distance. In sports performance, speed is composed of three factors:

- ☑ the latency time of the motor reaction
- ☑ the speed of the unique movement
- ☑ the frequency of the movement

The speed of movement depends on the degree of general and specific coordination of the athlete.

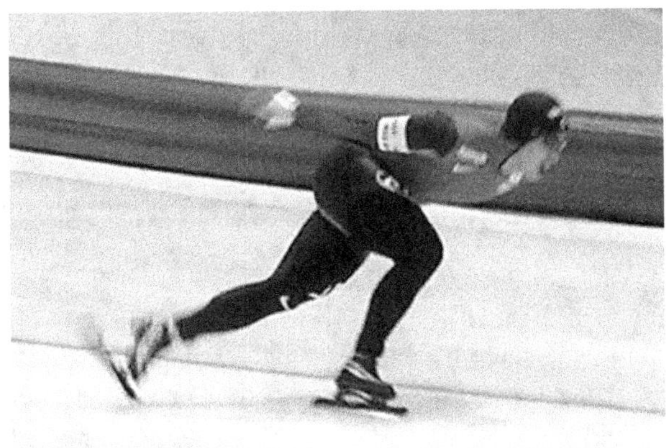

Speed comes in many forms:
- ☞ **Reaction** speed
- ☞ **Execution** speed
- ☞ **Repetition** speed
- ☞ **Movement** speed
- ☞ **Acceleration** speed

Speed, with strength and power, form together a set of parameters which allow performing actions at a maximal intensity. These two factors are part of the physical qualities of a sports complemented by the flexibility, coordination or address that involve specific skills as well as each sport.

The development of speed depends on several factors:

1. The **analyzers** operating state (visual, auditory, kinesthetic) in the direction of the sharpness, the fineness and accuracy of these analyzers.

2. The **capacity of analysis and synthesis** within the cerebral cortex

3. **The driving speed of the nerve impulse** to and from the muscles

4. **The attention** and sports concentration, which depends on the motivation and the age of the athlete

5. The type of innervation at the neuromuscular junction: for speed, it is the innervation by large alpha motor neurons that transmit rapid nerve impulse.

6. The **quality** and **type of muscle fibers** and **energy processes** that support the effort

7. The **muscle contraction speed** is determined mainly by the appearance of nerve innervation excitation and the type innervation, but also the type of muscle fiber.

8. The **joints mobility** and **muscle elasticity** that increase range and movement and promote movement efficiency

9. The **level of preparedness**

10. **The** athlete's **age** and **gender**

The development of speed depends on the relationship between the development of strength, the execution of movements' improvement and the technical functionality and plasticity of the nervous system.

Explosive strength

This factor, which influences athletic performance, represents the ability to produce a significant effort for a very short time (from 0 to 15 seconds). The explosive strength is ensured by the anaerobic alactic system.

We chose to treat the explosive strength (or "explosion" here) separately because of its importance in athletic performance. This capability is directly influenced by strength and speed. A balanced development of both strength and speed parameters generates a maximum "explosion" which is very important in some sports games where muscle energy and energy reserves are used to their maximum capacity to produce a quick and efficient explosion during a short time.

Other factors can come into action for the performance achieved by an athlete, especially those concerning the specific technique depending on the sport, but also the socio-psychological abilities of the individual. These are represented by the cognitive skills enabling one to understand and process information, but also their needed analysis to optimize performance. They manifest themselves particularly in intelligence, memory, analytical skills, etc. This category also includes affective capacities such as emotions, inclinations, feelings, etc.) which are real sources of energy for sports and manifest themselves through motivation, resistance to stress and pain, etc. Morale skills influence in equal measure the athlete's performance because they force her or him to master inner reactions during training and competitions.

Coordination

The "coordination" word includes address, intelligence, precision, finesse, grace, balance, stability and represents the ability of an individual to learn and quickly combine new movements in order to perform smooth and effective movements within a given time, with a low energy consumption level.

Coordination is influenced by several factors:

☞ The senses' operating state (visual, auditory, kinesthetic). The sensations' perception accuracy affects the precision of given orders and responses.

☞ The brain's ability to **select the information and react quickly.**

☞ The **plasticity of the cerebral cortex.**

☞ The short- and long-term **memory**
☞ **Quick and creative thinking**
☞ **Previous locomotion experience**
☞ The **joints mobility** and **muscle elasticity**
☞ **The athlete's age** and **gender**

Coordination can be trained in several ways, depending on the age and the specificity of the practiced sport, but it is a skill that is genetically determined, so that some athletes are "predestined" from birth to practice a particular sport.

Coordination manifests in two ways:

☑ Overall coordination
☑ Specific coordination (developed according to the discipline)

Coordination, unlike other qualities, develops from the youngest ages and continues to improve until maturity.

Mobility

Mobility is defined as the ability to carry large amplitude movements gracefully, harmony and low power consumption. It involves muscle elasticity and joint mobility and is considered a quality of musculo-articular device.

Mobility is influenced by several factors:

☞ **Joint type**: there are fixed, mobile and semi-mobile joints. Depending on the specific joints entrained within a given motion, mobility may be more or less important. In addition, the mobility of a same articulation differs from one individual to another.

☞ **Muscle mass**. It is considered that muscle hypertrophy limits movement, not because of the importance of the mass resulting from the increase in strength, but rather because of muscle stiffness. You can increase your muscle mass by force, but simultaneously with other broader movements that do not decrease muscle elasticity.

☞ **Muscle tone** and **relaxation capacity**. Increasing muscle tone reduces the ability to relax and stretch the muscle by increasing the intrinsic strength limit mobility in motion and, implicitly, performance. Insufficient coordination of neural processes that regulate the tension and relaxation of muscles negatively affects the level of mobility.

☞ **Muscle elasticity** and ligaments. The elasticity of tendons, ligaments and muscles are the most important factors affecting joint mobility.

☞ **Other factors**: fatigue, room temperature, age, gender, etc.

Mobility has two forms of expression:

1. **active** mobility, resulting in muscle demonstration (unassisted)

2. **passive** mobility, achieved with external forces (partner or training unit)

Mobility exercises have an important place during the warm-up and recovery phase after exercise. The best-known mobility exercises are those kind of **stretching**, which involve maintaining a certain position of a segment for a short period of time to gradually stretch a muscle and prepare it for a specific effort to which it will be submitted.

Indices to be considered for athletes

In many sports, success is influenced by the size and shape of the athlete. In some it is important to be sturdy and strong, in others large and slender or short and crisp. Acquiring the necessary physical capabilities for your chosen sport is also based on the gene pool available to you and can help you more in certain sports.

In any case, some of the factors influencing sports performance can be "manipulated" through diet and workouts. Many athletes decide at some point in their careers to change their level of body mass, muscle mass and body fat, and sometimes all at once.

Principles of the human body change in size / weight

Changing the energy balance in order to lose or gain body tissue can be done by changing the energy consumption or energy intake through diet or the combination of both. To promote muscle development, one must adapt training both in duration and intensity as well as frequency by harmonizing them with adequate food.

1. Body mass index

Body mass index (**BMI**), also known as Quetelet index, after the name of its Belgian inventor, is a quantity engineered to estimate the build of a person. It is calculated according to the size and body mass of the person.

The calculation of the body mass index according to the WHO (World Health Organization) is the result of the division of the weight by the square of height. It is the same for women as for men, whether they are athletes or not.

However, BMI is not calculated in the same way for major sports because it does not separate fat weight and muscle mass. To better understand the concept, a man's considered normal weight would have a BMI between 20 and 25. However, for athletes, this index can be greater than 25 because muscle mass is much more developed than normal. They are then considered as being obese according to the BMI grid. Massive athletes such as bodybuilders can even exceed a BMI of 30, which means "obesity"; that is obviously not the case for either the first or the second category.

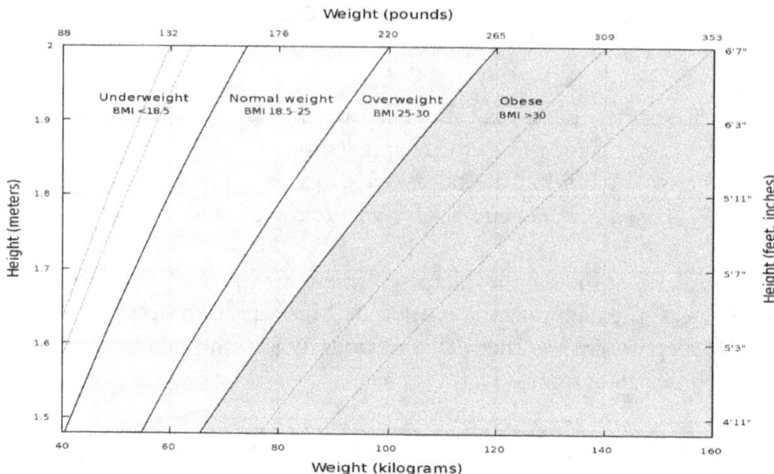

Although BMI is very important and is the first step to know when we reach an excessive weight, it is not enough to consider it as a single criterion. It may not accurately indicate the athlete's quality of life or functionality and cannot fully predict associated risks. For example, athletes who have the same body mass index may have fat percentage distributed differently, as well as other athletes with the same percentage of fat may have a different body mass index.

As a consequence, BMI is not applicable "as such" to athletes who have to find their equilibrium weight by taking into account muscle mass. More important for athletes is to primarily eliminate fat by keeping only muscles.

2. Fat rate and athlete's performance

The analysis of the body composition is used to monitor the effects of exercise on the active mass and adipose tissue. Athletes who lose weight through a restrictive diet because they exceed the requirements of a competition category may lose as much or even more active mass than fat. Sometimes, although the diet is associated with physical exercise, body weight might not change immediately, but we can see changes within body composition - in the direction of decreasing body fat and increasing active mass.

The human body is composed of fat and non-fat. The fat consists of essential fatty acids (the bone marrow, heart, lung, liver, spleen, kidney, central nervous system) and fat deposition (accumulated in the adipose tissue that is located around organs and in the subcutaneous regions).

The proportion of subcutaneous adipose tissue and internal fat is not the same for all athletes and can vary throughout life and at different stages of the preparation, for example in the phase before and during the competition when it is the least. Lean body mass is the weight of muscles, bones, ligaments, tendons, internal organs, teeth. Muscle tissue (muscle mass) is the body component that receives the strongest variations from the lean body mass (active material). The active mass is the one involved in the effort, and excess body fat has negative effects on health.

A certain percentage of fat is absolutely necessary to maintain health. Essential fatty acids are essential to the proper functioning of the body, and women have a higher percentage of essential fat than men.

The body fat level of athletes is considered a determining factor in the performance. This index is expressed as a percentage, in order to estimate the proportion of adipose tissue of a person.

Fat has a great potential for energy production. However, all body fat types are not available as "fuel". The fat percentage in athletes is not the same as in people with normal physical activity. This optimum value depends on the sporting activity practiced.

In athletes' bodies, the body fat percentage should not be interpreted independently, but in relation to her/his profile which incorporates changes in body mass index, weight, size, sex and the discipline practiced. It should not fall below a lower limit of fatness, to avoid exposure to health problems, and at the same time a loss of performance. This minimum limit is different for sportsmen and women and also varies depending on the discipline: for men it is advised to stay between 5 and 6%, while for women the range is wider between 12 and 16%.

The influence of a particular sport discipline consists in the kind of effort and energy metabolism needed for its practice (endurance, strength, speed).

There is no universal standard that applies to all athletes, especially as other individual factors come into play to sports performance.

Recommendations for optimal body fat levels are wide enough to allow covering all disciplines:
☞ Recommended BMI for male athletes is between 9 and 13%
☞ Advised BMI for female athletes varies between 12 and 23% even up to 28% depending on the discipline.

3. The ideal weight

The "ideal weight" is the average weight in which an athlete is in its best performance conditions. It depends on several factors such as the constitution of the sports (height, weight, frame), but also sex and the physical demands of his sport. For distance running a slim figure is ideal, while for a race weight is more important than size.

In order to determine the ideal weight we must take into account gender, age, height, body composition which is characterized by bone mass, fat mass, muscle mass, etc.

In some sports such as boxing, judo, wrestling, weightlifting, competition is organized by weight classes. In order to maintain its performance in its domain, the athlete must watch his diet carefully. It may also choose to change the category by adjusting its weight. However, remember that if you find yourself in this situation, it is recommended to do so under the advice and supervision of a professional sports nutritionist.

Warning! The body mass index does not calculate the ideal weight of an athlete, but a health risk. This is why it is applicable to any person. We must not confuse both notions!

In some sports, weight maintenance is very important; gymnasts for instance, who with a few extra grams completely change one's exercise when one's center of gravity is changed, creating variations within important factors such as angles, inertia, stability, etc. This is why it is very important to control this factor permanently if you want performance. Although some athletes have a large body mass, it is essential that this mass is as high as the active muscle mass rather than body fat percentage.

So, what to remember is that the ideal weight is one in which you, as an athlete, feel in harmony with your body and your mind. You can reach this weight through a balanced diet. If you are top athlete, the ideal weight is the one that represents the best compromise between a minimum of fat tissue within body and optimal physical strength.

Genetics and sports performance

If for a long time, it was considered that the will, drive and perseverance were the only factors influencing sports performance, scientists have shown that other parameters also intervened in this performance level as we have seen in previous chapters.

We know there are a number of differences between populations regarding sports performance. For example, in 2002, the Boston Marathon Kenyans were present 14 athletes, 13 of them (93%) ranked in the top 25 places. By contrast, among 1.122 Canadian athletes, only one ranked in the top 25. The huge disparity between the participating ethnic groups can mean an innate ability of the African people to run long distances. Today it is known with certainty that there is a hereditary component for an athlete in the way of interacting with environmental factors, in this case: training.

Genetics also seems to have a significant part in the performance of athletes.

Today we know that there are about 200 genes correlated with athletic performance. In addition, there are 16 mitochondrial genes whose variants appear to have a significant influence on sport activity.

Scientists have identified genes that can improve sports performance. The following summarizes some examples of genes and their effects on sports performance:

The **ACTN3** gene that acts on fast muscle fibers and whose studies (see here an article published in 2003 by Am J Hum Genet on *US National Library of Medicine National Institutes of Health* https://www.ncbi.nlm.nih.gov/pmc/articles/PMC1180686/) showed it could affect the sprint performance and, in its mutated variant, influences athletes' endurance. However, according to experts, the influence of ACTN3 on physical capacities reveals its importance among top athletes.

The **ACE** gene produces a protein that plays a role in the regulation of blood flow and, according to the present variant, the athlete will be most suitable for an endurance activity.

The **ADRB2** gene produces epinephrine, affecting blood glucose and blood circulation. Studies have shown that the **Gln27** variant is associated with successful endurance; his presence was reported in the most elite athletes in endurance sports. Good nutrition, appropriate exercise and nutritional supplements can play an important role in the management of this impact.

The **CNTF** gene produces a nerve growth factor that acts as a communicator between cells and is associated with muscle strength.

The **CRP** gene can significantly increase during exercise. It can affect the levels of proteins in the blood in response to exercise and lead to an overall decrease of endurance. A balanced diet can correct the negative impact of high levels of CRP. Carbohydrate consumption of a certain type, increasing the quantity and the introduction of fiber has shown a positive effect on maintaining a low level of CRP in the blood during exercise.

The **NOS3** gene produces an important enzyme for the state of blood vessels.

The **PPARGC1A** gene plays a key role in the energy balance involved in the slow-twitch muscle fibers in training.

The **VDR** gene encodes the protein receptor for vitamin D, a protein involved in many processes in the body. It is associated with an increase in strength and muscle mass.

Another example is the cellular receptor of **erythropoietin** which is a hormone involving an increased number of red blood cells. A genetic mutation therefore enables a superior production of red blood cells than average and thus improves oxygen supply to the muscle by increasing athletes' endurance.

Genetics also influences the size of people, which is essential in specific sports like basketball for example.

Genes also appear to play a role in the length of the Achilles heel, which is very important for athletes practicing high jump.

A mutation of the **HFE** gene on human chromosome 6 decreases the production of hepcidin and increases the availability of iron for the production of a greater amount of red blood cells and muscle. This iron will not be stored, unlike what happens in people with the mutation and who do not practice sports intensively. Athletes with this mutation are more effective in manifesting differently depending on the discipline and cross country skiing, skiers will synthesize more hemoglobin in altitude than other competitors, while in judo there will be an advantage in faster regeneration of muscle cells.

According to research and studies done so far, it seems rare that only a single gene is involved in sports performance. It is rather a set of genes that show their potential within a particular environment, with specific training and a tailored diet. It is important not to overlook all the other factors that are essential to determine the level of performance of an athlete.

Role of hydration in sports performance

The human body is not a closed system and every day water losses through urine, perspiration, respiration, etc. must be compensated by adequate and regular water supply. Human body is over 50% water and needs on average 2 to 3 liters per day to compensate for these losses, but also for all reactions which it belongs. Body water needs are covered for more than half by drinks such as water, fruit juices, coffee, tea, milk, etc. and the rest from food. In the case of male and female athletes, hydration is very important for the proper functioning of the body. So if you play a sport aiming performance, be aware that uncompensated losses of water affect your performance. As a consequence, you really have to attach a particular importance to hydration during workouts, competitions and even in everyday life. A strong dehydration during exercise can cause discomfort that can even lead to death.

For athletes, the greatest loss of water during sport practice comes from sweating. It can reach several liters per hour in case of intense effort. Poor hydration can cause a decline in your performance and even tendonitis, as well as other conditions such as kidney stones that can form, following the reduction of irrigation kidney.

Hydration participates in cooling the body during intense physical activity, and if it is not properly secured, this absence can cause a thermal shock in the form of heat stroke. This phenomenon involves the rise of body temperature exceeding a critical threshold and is accompanied by a rapid heart rate, headaches, a drop in blood pressure and other symptoms. It can become serious and lead to neurological sequelae or death.

If you are an endurance athlete, you need to drink regularly before, during and after exercise in order to maintain optimum hydration of your body. You can also drink an isotonic energy drink that can bring to your system essential nutrients especially if your exercise lasts longer than one hour. These sports drinks are specifically designed to provide the body of the athlete with what he lost during intense physical activity, such as simple carbohydrates and minerals which are essential to the proper functioning of the body. After exercise, you enter the recovery phase, but you have to remain hydrated to compensate for losses of water and minerals. A mineralizing and isotonic (sports) drink can help replace these items.

The daily fluids needs vary by sport (individual variation), type and intensity of physical effort. Liquid losses are genetically determined and **directly proportional** to:

- ☑ **body surface area:** fluid loss increases with the increase of the body surface
- ☑ the **degree of physical preparation** (fitness): affects the composition and the volume of fluid loss, so for a trained athlete, perspiration occurs early in a volume higher but diluted (low sodium chloride NaCl)
- ☑ the **environment:** a humid environment and a high temperature accelerates the loss of liquids. Similarly, altitude training intensifies loss of fluid.
- ☑ **intensity** of training: endurance sports require a higher and more frequent consumption of fluids.

On average, a sedentary adult needs about 2.5 liters of water per day from food and liquids to replace the water lost through urine and respiration. For an athlete, these losses are added to the water loss due to perspiration.

The Hydration Guide during exercise of the American College of Sports Medicine (ACSM) recommends:

- ☞ adequate hydration 24 hours before the exercise
- ☞ a consumption of 400 to 600 ml of liquid two hours before training
- ☞ a consumption of 150 to 350 ml of fluid every 15-20 minutes during exercise.

Hydration should be maintained at optimal parameters, particularly if the athlete is exposed to high ambient temperatures and high humidity. In these cases, and especially if the sport implies endurance, loss of fluids and electrolytes through sweating can lead to lower body temperature to levels that cause certain symptoms. During an intense and prolonged exercise, some athletes can lose up to 2.7 to 3.6 kg per hour due to loss of water and electrolytes. If the training lasts for more than an hour, rehydration solution must be added.

The substances recommended in rehydration solutions are:

- ☑ **carbohydrates** (Carbohydrates) 30-100 mg / liter
- ☑ **sodium** (Na) 1100 mg / liter
- ☑ **osmolarity** less than 500 milliosmols.

Optional ingredients are:

- ➤ Chlorine 1500 mg / liter maximum
- ➤ Potassium 225 mg / liter maximum
- ➤ Magnesium 100 mg / liter maximum
- ➤ Calcium 225 mg / liter maximum

These drinks can be prepared or can be purchased in the form of isotonic (sports) drinks. Only rehydration drinks containing carbohydrates and electrolytes may improve cognitive processes during exercise and motor skills. The consumption of carbohydrates can be beneficial to support intense and very intense exercise lasting an hour or more, and less intense exercise but with a long duration. It has been shown that 30-60 g/h of carbohydrates represent the optimal amount to maintain blood sugar levels and support physical effort.

To understand the process, you have to know that in case of dehydration, the volume of water contained in the blood plasma is reduced, blood thickens and the heart has to make more effort to pump up vessels. The blood circulation in the capillaries becomes more and more difficult and the level of oxygen and nutrients feeding the muscle will decrease as well as the ability to eliminate muscle toxins. The heart will be forced to increase his pace to maintain blood pressure. Thus, your performance will decrease and there will be a 10% decline in your physical abilities for a loss of 1% of your weight in water.

Hydration is not only important during exercise but it is necessary during the days before the scheduled sports activity or competition to help maintain the water balance of the body. If you want to know your water needs during exercise you can do a simple test: weigh yourself before and after a workout while taking into consideration the amount of water that you drank during the activity. This simple test will let you know your water needs during training. Temperature and climate conditions can also impact the calculation and therefore when it is hot, you will have the greatest needs for losses through perspiration will also be more important during exercise. It is recommended to split your water intake throughout the effort, to avoid bloating. The best reaction is to drink 100 to 200 ml of water every 15 to 20 minutes. It is also important to know that drinking excess water can lead to hyponatremia. However, this happens very rarely and is caused by cells over hydration that led to the dissolution of sodium in the blood. This condition can cause symptoms such as nausea, vomiting, drowsiness and even breathing difficulty and in extreme cases, seizures, loss of consciousness, which can lead to death. It is also important to know that excess drinking can lead to hyponatremia. However, this happens very rarely and is caused by cells over hydration that leads to the dissolution of sodium in the blood. This condition can cause symptoms such as nausea, vomiting, drowsy and even difficulty breathing and in extreme cases, seizures, loss of consciousness, which can lead to death.

Sports drinks

Sports drinks are beverages specially designed for rehydration. They contain electrolytes (sodium chloride, magnesium, potassium) and carbohydrates. The amount of carbohydrate is not high, being calculated in such a way to provide you with sufficient energy for the effort.

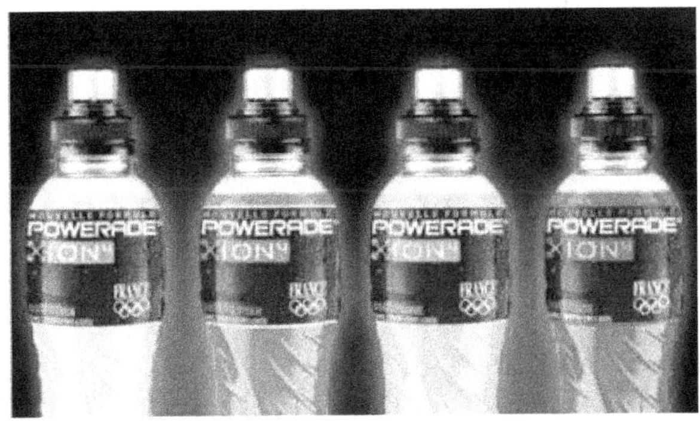

There are 3 types of sports drinks which differ in their absorption rate into the bloodstream:

hypotonic	isotonic	hypertonic
Fewer elements dissolved in the blood	The same number of elements dissolved in the blood	More elements dissolved in the solution in the blood
Fast water absorption	Maximum absorption rate	This type of drink provides less rehydration
Still water, mineral water, fruit or herbal tea, very diluted natural juices, mineral and vitamin drinks	Fruit juice mix, isotonic drinks, mineral and vitamin drinks with a higher concentration	Undiluted natural juices, lemonade, iced tea, energy drinks
This type of beverage is suitable for rapid rehydration	This type of drink is suitable before and after exercise to relieve mineral loss and maintain blood volume and blood sugar.	To boost or reload reserves. Not only suitable for rehydration, as short-term body fluids are absorbed to bring the components of the drink consumed at the same concentration as blood.

For physical efforts that last **less than one hour**, fluid loss can be compensated by hypotonic drinks. These should be made **without alcohol, nor caffeine or sugar**. So you can use mineral water, much diluted fruit juice in a ratio of 1: 2 or a vitamin mineral drink.

In the case of **extreme physical exertion**, which is accompanied by a large loss of fluids through sweating, and for activities that last **more than one hour**, adequate hydration is necessary, with drinks that can compensate for mineral losses and carbohydrates. In this case, it is essential to use **hypotonic or isotonic drinks**. For the energy contained in blood to be available for longer periods so that the pancreas must not release a large amount of insulin, it is necessary to consume complex carbohydrates. Carbohydrates in the form of fructose are suitable in a proportion of one third of the total amount of carbohydrates to prevent the risk of diarrhea.

In the case of **endurance sports** in times of high heats, **continuous** fluid intake is **essential** for the body. During competition, while struggling with other competitors, it is easy to forget the regular supply of the body with liquids. To avoid this problem you may, for example, set your watch to beep every 15 minutes. This way you will not forget to drink and will ensure proper hydration, which will increase your performance. If, during a competition, you start drinking when the feeling of thirst comes, know that it is already too late. The athlete does not drink during competition to quench his thirst, but to keep his exercise capacity at the highest possible level.

A **good isotonic drink** should offset the loss of body fluids due to sweating during exercise, but also replace lost minerals through sweat while being a source of energy thanks to its carbohydrate content. It is preferable for it to have a low carbohydrate rate from fructose (to prevent onset of diarrhea) and have a pleasant taste.

Caution, do not confuse sports (isotonic) drinks with energy drinks that are not at all the same thing and do not have all the same properties. You can find more details in the "Food Supplements" section. Please read carefully the labels of drinks you buy so you cannot get "fooled" by marketing labels that may easily induce confusion.

In conclusion, the proper management of the water balance of the body is a key optimization of athletic performance.

Role of nutrition in sports performance

Diet greatly influences the performance of the athlete and the foods you eat both before and during or after training and during competitions will determine your athletic performance. Athletes should be aware of their nutritional goals and how to select a real specific dietary strategy to achieve these objectives. The diet can have a big impact on training and competition and a good diet will help support intensive workouts while reducing the risk of injury or illness.

Making the right food choices can also produce positive adjustments in muscle and other tissues in response to stimulation in training. Athletes are different and there is no universal diet that meets the needs of all. People also change throughout the season and athletes must learn to be flexible in order to adapt to these changes.

Acquiring the optimal amount of energy to stay in shape, healthy and efficient is essential. Too much energy and body fat increases, too little and performance decreases along with the risk of the occurrence of accidents or illnesses.

Carbohydrates are key nutrients for energy supply, but the need for carbohydrates depends in particular on the length and intensity of workouts. Peopole must therefore adapt their diet based on several parameters we will help you to know and master in this chapter and those that follow.

Athletes should know the right sources of carbohydrates and adopt them in their diet and at the same time learn to avoid foods that can harm their shape and health.

Foods which are rich in protein are important for building and repairing muscles, but the daily diet can provide adequate protein level without the need for supplementation. The timing and type of protein are just as important as the amount of protein in the diet. Even vegetarian diets - if they are well chosen - can provide protein needs of an athlete. A varied diet rich in nutrients provides enough energy for the needs of an athlete and should be mainly composed of vegetables, fruits, legumes, cereals and their complete derivatives, lean meats, quality oils and dairy products. A healthy and balanced diet provides sufficient amounts of all vitamins and minerals, as well as essential fatty acids, which are requested for a good functioning of an athlete's organism: the foundation of performance.

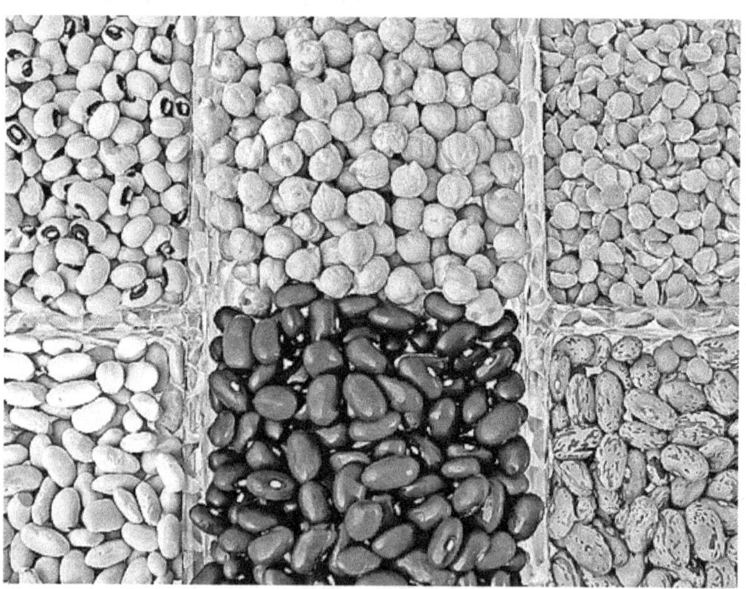

A **balanced diet** at every meal and during training has many benefits for athletes not only by securing the necessary inputs of nutrients, but also allowing it to greatly reduce potential injuries and other ailments. It also allows him/her to recover better after exercise and stabilize weight.

For an athlete, it is important to meet the nutritional needs because it allows the body to move in an optimum nutritional environment for sports performance.

Each sportsperson has specific nutritional needs that are determined based on several parameters such as age, sex, height, weight, genetic heritage, but also the sport practiced and the level of effort during training. Nevertheless, it is possible to create a profile of these needs both in terms of energy, as well as macro- and micronutrients inputs. If you want a specific analysis for your nutritional needs, we recommend that you meet with a sports nutrition specialist to adjust your diet to the type of sport you practice, taking into account the frequency and intensity of your workouts.

As you have understood from the previous chapter, proper hydration is also essential to athletic performance. Appropriate fluid intake before, during and after physical activity is vital, especially in hot climates. Replacement of salt is essential when losses by sweating are great, but these needs vary from one athlete to another.

You will find in this section - and the following - information that will help you make informed choices to ensure your nutritional needs in different situations. Obviously, this guide is not a substitute for individual recommendations received from a qualified professional in sports nutrition, but you may consider it as "handy" and practical foundation for a suitable nutrition for athletes aiming performance.

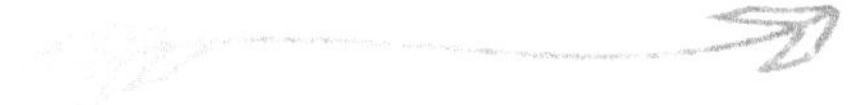

Energy needs of the athlete

The energy needs of an athlete are different from those of a sedentary person or with a moderate physical activity, as you can easily imagine. These needs consist of several factors, including metabolic energy basic needs. These are necessary for cell maintenance, temperature control, proper functioning of the immune system, growth, but also to support regular and often intense physical activity.

The energy used in one of these processes is not available for others. It is for this reason that diet plays an important role as it will provide enough energy to meet the needs of all essential body functions. Physical activity and in the case of an athlete, the intensity, duration and frequency of training sessions and competitions will play a vital role in determining its daily energy needs.

When the energy of daily intake from food and concretized in carbohydrates, fats and proteins, are equivalent to the energy consumption, the sport is said to be in **"energy balance."** The formula is:

Energy balance = energy intake - energy consumption

For an athlete, it is crucial to meet the nutritional needs, which are much greater than for a person with normal physical activity. This coverage allows the body to move in an optimum nutritional environment for sports performance.

Energy availability

Energy availability is a concept that represents the energy left to the body to allow metabolic functions run correctly except those directly related to the actual physical activity. This availability is calculated as the difference between energy intake induced by food and energy costs caused by exercise. It must be maintained for a sportsperson to 30 kcal per kg body weight per day. This is a threshold below which the athlete can not only lose its performance, but even lead to chronic energy deficiency that can harm health, especially in case of repeated deficits.

Carbohydrates

The carbohydrate needs vary greatly from one athlete to another, but also the type and intensity of the workout you do. They may be established by a nutritionist, but if you want to get an idea of the order of measurement, they are usually between 3 and 10 g / kg / day. So if you weigh 75 kg, you will need between 225 g and 750 g of carbohydrates per day. This range is quite wide because it depends a lot on the sport you practice.

Lipids

Lipids needs are also big thanks to their multiple roles, not only in terms of energy but also at structural and functional levels. Essential fatty acids are vital in the metabolism of sports. As for carbohydrates, recommendations vary from one athlete to another, but experts advise to have food rations with a minimum of 25% fat.

Proteins

In terms of protein requirements, they are mainly determined by the type of sport you practice. If you practice a discipline that involves endurance, your protein needs are between 1.2 and 1.4 g / kg body weight / day, whereas if your sport is focused on strength, you will need more protein: between 1.3 and 1.5 g / kg / day. These needs may be higher while taking muscle mass and reach up to 2 g / kg / day. In all cases, it is not advisable to exceed 2.5 g / kg / day. Be careful not to consume large amounts of protein for long periods because it can affect not only your performance but even harm your health.

Vitamins and minerals

Vitamins and minerals play an essential role in all physiological mechanisms. As an athlete, it is important to ensure a balanced diet that covers the needs of vitamins and minerals, especially as you have higher needs than an average person who does not practice sports performance. We advise you to eat more foods with high nutrient density, thus being richer in micronutrients in relation to their energy intake.

Eat fruits and vegetables, but also dairy products low in fat and sugars, eggs, fish and seafood, unrefined carbohydrates like pasta to wholegrain cereals, whole meal bread and cereals, brown rice, legumes such as lentils, chickpeas, white beans, nuts such as walnuts, hazelnuts, almonds.

Avoid sausages and other processed meat products, too sweet and savory products, soft drinks, fatty meats and dairy products that contain too much fat and added sugar.

If you want to cover your nutritional needs, you can do this through a balanced diet accompanied by adequate hydration. Know that your nutritional approach should be part of a long-term process if you want to see real results.

The increase in performance is gradual - so be patient - but you will also find that you will be less prone to accidents such as injuries, tendonitis and sprains.

Example of a daily diet

A **healthy and balanced diet for a sportsperson** must include:

1. A **hearty breakfast**, the first meal of the day which is very important for your shape. For example it may be composed with:

- ☑ a fresh glass of juice pressed with the fibers – a smoothie without adding sugar,
- ☑ 3 slices of whole meal bread or 5 full grain crackers,
- ☑ little or no butter with pure fruit jam (it has a lot of carbohydrates so eat according to your carbohydrate needs),

Opt for unsweetened breakfast with hummus and other spreads homemade (with eggplants, eggs, peas, lentils, etc.) with extra-virgin olive oil. You can also eat canned sardines (rich in calcium) or mackerel - natural or with olive oil.

- ☑ A hot drink such as milk, coffee or tea. It is better not to mix them because digestion will be disrupted,
- ☑ Natural yoghurt with little fat or soy,
- ☑ A fruit: kiwi, banana, grapes, apple, orange, etc.

2. For **a balanced meal for lunch** here the ideal composition:

- ☑ A serving of fresh or cooked vegetables. You can either eat a salad (with a tablespoon of canola oil or olive seasoning and lemon juice) or as an accompaniment to meat;
- ☑ A source of protein such as meat food, preferably as thin as poultry. Fatty fish like salmon, sardines and mackerel are also excellent sources of protein and essential fatty acids. You can also eat seafood or eggs. Of course, do not eat it all at once but choose the protein sources you prefer :-);
- ☑ A portion of starchy foods like pasta or rice complete, pulses such as lentils, white or red beans, chick-peas, cornmeal form of polenta, but also potatoes. For best results, in the case of potatoes, you have to eat in the same time cooked green vegetables like green beans, spinach, broccoli, cabbage, chard, eggplant, zucchini, leeks, fennel, peas, etc.
- ☑ You can also eat 2-3 slices of whole meal bread or cereal depending on the load of your workout for the day;

☑ A dairy product such as soft cheese type Camembert or goat cheese, Saintt Nectaire. Caution: it must be a small portion and do not eat at all meals (no more than 4 times per week), plain yogurt or cottage cheese;

☑ A fresh fruit: apples, peaches, kiwi;

☑ A dessert if you want, but not more than 3 times a week.

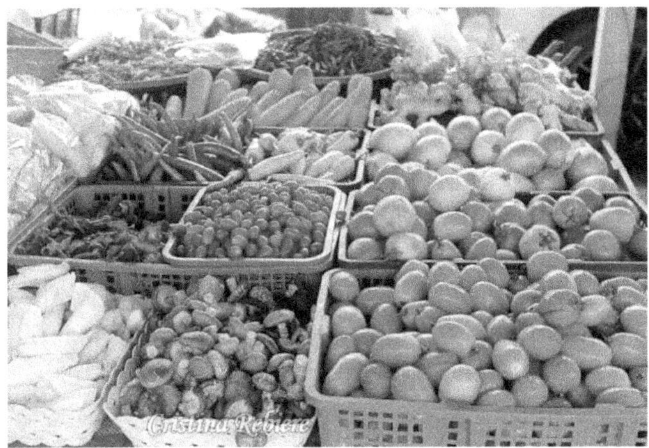

3. The recommended **dinner** is almost the same as a lunch but you can eat a soup of greens, a plate of vegetables with a third of starchy food and two thirds of cooked green vegetables. Prefer meat to seafood for better digestion. For the dairy product, prefer natural yoghurt instead of cheese that promotes weight gain. If you long for a dessert, take a fruit compote that is more digestible than a fresh fruit.

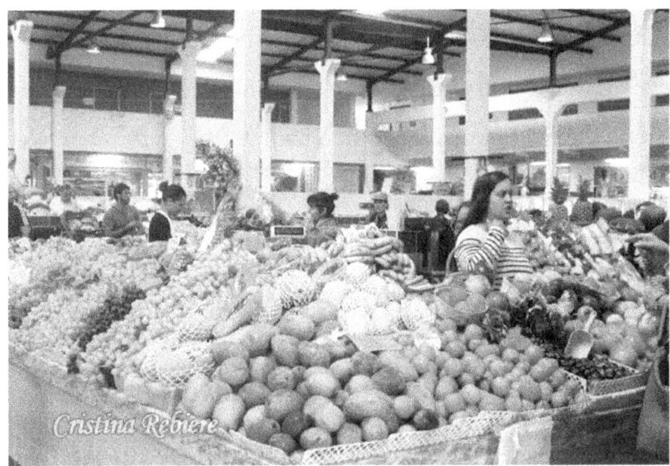

4. You may – or will even have to - take one or more **snacks** depending on your training **to properly distribute food intake over the day**. This snack can be a fruit (strawberries, raspberries, cherries, apples or pears with their skin). You can add natural yogurt without sugar or a cereal bar with a percentage of fat less than 10% or 3-4 whole grain crackers.

How to calculate your energy needs?

It is not easy to accurately calculate your energy needs, but this parameter is one that influences your sports performance. It is for this reason that even a rough estimate is better than to completely ignore your energy needs and supply yourself "randomly" because it is more difficult to fill the gaps or clear excess thereafter. You must adjust your diet according to the frequency and intensity of your workouts.

The formula for calculating the energy needs of a person is as follows:

Energy requirements (ER) = Basal Metabolic Rate (BR) x activity factor (AF)

The activity factor (AF) has been determined by the degree of activity of a person:

- ☑ sedentary ⇒ AF = 1.35
- ☑ weakly active ⇒ AF = 1.55
- ☑ active ⇒ AF = 1.75
- ☑ very active ⇒ AF = 1.95

The formula of basal metabolism is different according to sex, age, size and weight of the person.

You can find several options on the Wikipedia page for the calculation of basic metabolism. The best known is the **formula of Harris and Benedict** was recalculated by Roza Shizgal in 1984. As for women, the formula is as follows:

BM = 9.74 x weight in kg + 172.9 x height in m - 4.73 x age + 667

And for the men:

BM = 13.7 x weight in kg + 492.3 x height in m - 6.67 x age + 77.6

In the sport filed and even on the Wikipedia page in English, the given information is not the same...

ASTUCE To easily calculate your needs, we suggest using the calculator on this website: http://www.globalrph.com/harris-benedict-equation.htm which applies the formula Harris and Benedict.

Basic metabolism formula for a **woman**:

BM = 655.1 + (9.563 x weight in kg) + (1.850 x height in cm) - (4.676 x age in years)

Basic metabolism formula for a **man**:

BM = 66.47 + (13.75 x weight in kg) + (5.003 x height in cm) - (6.755 x age in years)

Example calculation of the energy requirements for a 32 years old woman, measuring 1.70 m and weighing 60 kg with an intense activity (in an endurance sport for example):

AF = 1.75 for intensive training of 2 hours, 3 times a week

BM = 655 + (9.56 x 60) + (1.85 x 170) - (4.67 x 32) – 655 + 573.6 + 314.5 - 149.4 = 1592 kcal

So the daily energy requirements of this woman will be:
ER = 1592 x 1.70 = 2706 kcal per day
At these energy needs must be added liquids needs to ensure proper hydration: 2 liters a day without training and up to 3.5 liters in the days with training.
Another relevant site to calculate your energy needs is here: http://www.calculator.net/bmr-calculator.html. You will get slightly different results, but they do not exceed one hundred kcal variation.

Recommended diet for endurance athletes

By physical endurance we understand cardiovascular, respiratory and muscular endurances. The heart and breathing function have to be able to provide sufficient oxygen to ensure the intensity of the effort. Upon prolonged effort in time, mostly muscle type 1 fibers are stimulated. The psychological factor plays an essential role in endurance because if you practice an endurance sport, you need a strong will and a moral resistance to fatigue in order to maintain the level of your performance during training and competition. Among the endurance sports there are foot races, marathons, bicycle races, cross country skiing, biathlon, triathlon, heptathlon, etc.

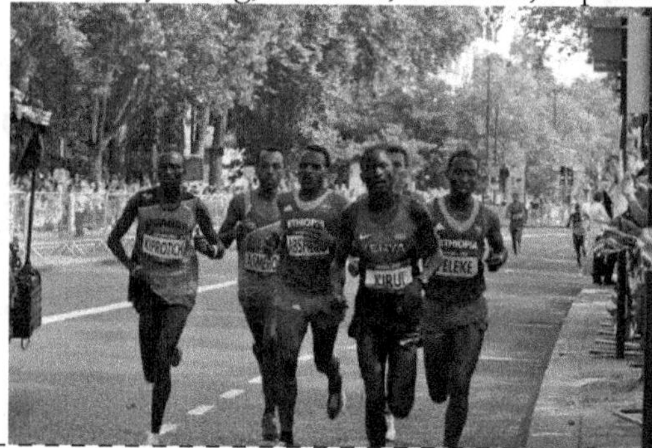

Basic principles of a diet adapted to endurance sport

If you are endurance sportsperson, as you probably already know, a balanced and well distributed food during the day are your main assets to optimize your performance in addition to proper training. It should allow you to support your body with the energy you need for your physical activities of the day. As we saw within the previous section, the ideal is to spread your food intake throughout the day in the form of three balanced meals and one or two snacks to fill the energy deficit induced by physical effort for your workouts. To get to maximize your athletic performance, know that it is important to take into account in addition to your nutritional needs, the quality of food you consume, their provenience, as well as their preparation mode which can influence their nutritional value.

The carbohydrate intake is more important for endurance athletes than in other sports because it is the carbohydrates that allow you to provide the energy needed for intense and prolonged physical exertion. During your intensive training, choose meals with low glycemic index and starchy foods such as pasta and brown rice, semolina wheat or corn.

It is advisable to vary the energy input between the training phases, especially depending on its load. To keep adequate energy availability, here are some helpful tips:

☞ Consume carbohydrates depending on your nutritional needs for the training phase (usually the level of these carbohydrates you need is moderate to high because you drop a lot of effort);

☞ Hydrate yourself properly during prolonged training sessions;

☞ To facilitate your recovery, consume nutrients after training as liquids or electrolytes for rehydration, carbohydrates, but also a source of high quality protein and an amount of 20 to 25 g to facilitate muscle adaptation.

The acid-base balance should be monitored as well, as it helps to preserve muscle mass and bone mass using calcium in an overly acidic environment, to maintain balance and can cause bone demineralization. To preserve this acid-base balance, eat as many acidifying foods, high in protein and sulfur amino acids, such as meat, fish, dairy products or eggs as those which are less acidifying like fruits, vegetables and grains. It is up to you to tailor your diet according to your preferences also because eating has to make you happy and should certainly not be a chore.

Nutrition before - during - and after exercise for the endurance athlete

Before exercise
If you are preparing for a competition, the diet can help you prepare your organization to optimize performance. Eat carbohydrates to meet your nutritional needs depending on the level of competition and workouts (consider the frequency and duration!). If for example you have an event that lasts more than 90 minutes, your carbohydrate load should not be considered for only the day of the competition, but also during the last 2 - 3 days before the race.
Food and beverages consumed before the sporting exercise must be digestible to not cause digestive disorders that could reduce athletic performance. It is recommended not to eat 2 to 3 hours before the start of the effort. It is also important to drink enough to maintain a good hydration.
Carbohydrates are important before exercise because they provide the "fuel", but also used after exercise to allow the body to replenish its glycogen stores. Nevertheless, limit foods which are high in fat or fiber to reduce the risk of gastrointestinal disorders during exercise.

During exercise
During the exercise, it is essential to prevent dehydration while limiting depletion of glycogen stores. The more intense is effort with a prolonged duration, the higher the water loss is important.

Weather conditions can also play an important role and should be taken into account. Excessive water loss affects the physical and mental performance of the athlete and that's why it must ensure adequate hydration needs during exercise.

For prolonged efforts beyond an hour, the consumption of a specific drink for the effort is necessary. It is the same during the competition days. The intake of carbohydrates during prolonged and intense sports activity increases endurance over time while maintaining performance.

The consumption of carbohydrates by a **special effort drink** must be done according to the athlete and the practiced sport, as well as in relation with the climatic conditions. For high energy demand periods, the drink should have a high concentration of carbohydrates (about 60 g/L). These carbohydrates are glucose type fructose and maltodextrin that ensure proper assimilation of the drink. On the contrary, if fluid intake is more important for the activity, then the concentration of carbohydrates will not exceed 30 to 40 g/L. A small amount of salt added to the drink can keep the water status longer, but should not exceed 1 to 1.2 g/L.

In addition to hydration, a contribution in the form of an energy bar or fruit paste is also recommended for endurance sport.

After the effort

After efforts spent during intense physical activity, **recovery** is an essential step in maintaining performance. The average sportsperson trains at least once a day and top athletes can even have multiple workouts per day. An adequate recovery between two training helps maintaining performance during the next workout. For competition, things are similar because several events can be linked and the athlete needs to know how to recover well in order to keep his/her abilities to the maximum level.

Recovery requires **good hydration** depending on the spent effort and be well above the water loss (1.5 times), restoration of glycogen stores and muscle recovery.

Some drinks rehydrate better in this recovery step such as milk that does not cause a significant increase in urine volume as water. However water rich in sodium is very effective for recovery.

To rebuild glycogen stores, the endurance athlete's diet should be adapted both in terms of foods from the time that they were taken. It is recommended that carbohydrate consumption to intervene quickly after exercise, so the amount of synthesized muscle glycogen will be greater. This is especially the case if the recovery period between sessions is less than 8 hours.

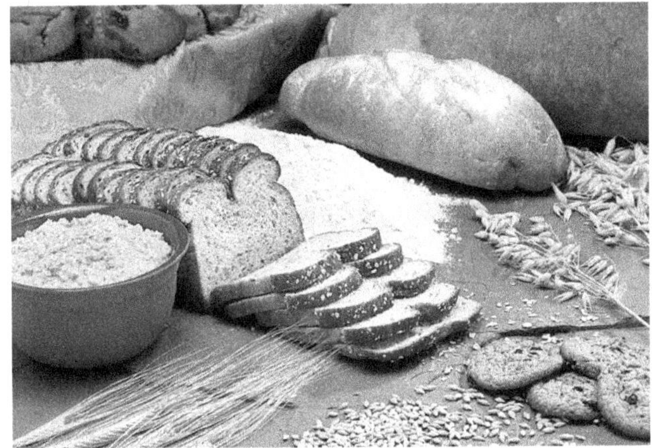

By studying glycogen re-synthesis during recovery, it appears that consumption of 20 to 30g of carbs every 15 minutes is optimal for athletes who have several sessions of physical effort. This carbohydrate intake can be embodied in a cereal bar, fruit juice briquette few slices of whole meal bread, a milk briquette. This contribution can be reduced if it is supplemented by a contribution of proteins that also optimizes glycogen re-synthesis, while ensuring the rebuilding of muscle fibers. This contribution can weigh from 20 to 25g. Milk is very suitable for this contribution.

Finally, a balanced meal rich in carbohydrates is recommended 2 or 3 hours after exercise.

Sample diet for endurance athletes

The diet of a sportsperson who practices an endurance sport is to be adapted to the frequency of workouts. Here is a sample daily diet to give you an idea of a balanced meal suitable for an endurance sport practiced by a woman.

Solid breakfast:

- ☑ 2 slices of whole meal bread or cereal or 4 complete rusks or cereals representing between 140 and 180 kcal and containing approximately 30 g of complex carbohydrates, 11 g protein and 1 g of lipids
- ☑ 50 g hummus representing 142 kcal, with 3 g of protein, between 4 and 5 g of carbohydrate, about 12 g of fat, more than 200 mg of sodium, 2.5 g of fibers
- ☑ 100 g oatmeal 60g carbohydrate with a low glycemic index and 12g protein

☑ 100 g of milk: 63 kcal; 3.2 g protein, 4.6 g carbohydrates, between 3 and 4 g of lipids

☑ Natural yoghurt with little fat: 47 kcal; 4 g of protein, 4 to 5 g carbohydrate, less than 1 g of lipids

☑ An orange: 47 kcal; 11.75 g carbohydrate, 940 mg of protein, 120 mg lipid

Breakfast one day without training

Food	kcal	carbohydrate g	protein g	fat g
2 slices bread, whole wheat, toasted	140	30	11	1
16 g natural peanut butter	100	3	4	8
1 cup skim milk, 0%	86	10	6.5	0.2

Breakfast one day with training

Food	kcal	carbohydrate g	protein g	fat g
total:	859			
2 slices bread, whole wheat, toasted	140	30	11	1
50 g hummus	142	4.5	3	12
1 cup skim milk, 0%	86	11	8.3	0.4
100 g oatmeal	368	60	14	6
5 g dried cranberries	15	4	0.05	0.07
1 apple	52	13.8	0.26	0.17
natural yoghurt, 0%	56	7.6	5.5	0.1

Morning snack: 1 fruit

Food	kcal	carbohydrate g	protein g	fat g
1 apple	52	13.8	0.26	0.17
1 fishing	36	11	0.7	0.09
1 banana	72.3	15.2	0.98	0.25

During workout, you need to add a cereal bar (representing more than 200 kcal) for example.

Food	kcal	carbohydrate g	protein g	fat g
total:	643			
100 g Salmon baked or grilled	171	0.49	24	7.5
wholewheat pasta	123	26	5.3	0.54
50 g lettuce 1 case with extra virgin olive oil	8 119	1.63	0.5	0.08 13.5
100 g cooked lentils	165	18.73	8.39	6.76
100 g blueberries	57	14.5	0.74	0.33

Afternoon snack:

Food	kcal 102	carbohydrate g	protein g	fat g
2 dates	46	12.4	0.4	0.06
1 yogurt, 0%	56	7.6	5.5	0.1

A second snack may be necessary during training.

Food	kcal	carbohydrate g	protein g	fat g
total:	328			
100 g beet salad	61	9.6	1.6	2.2
Rice 1 cup cooked whole wheat	214	44.4	5	1.7
Stewed Apples no Added Sugars	53	12	0	0

To know the nutritional value of foods you can use this website: https://www.fatsecret.fr/calories-nutrition/.

Of course, do not forget **hydration** before, during and after physical activity.

If you do the kcal math in our table while applying the formula we have given you to calculate energy requirements, you will see data changing depending on your weight and your gender.

This sample diet is only a reference model and like all reference examples are often less caloric. Why? Simply because energy requirements are influenced by other factors. In addition to the digestive and absorption mechanisms, it must be taken into account that the person also continues the energy absorption of the earlier meal / snack. The reference diet is rarely respected and the athlete must adapt according to their personal preferences and needs. There are people who eat less; others who need more, even if both are athletes in the same discipline, have the same age, height and weight. The ideal principle is to "listen" to your body because if you are hungry, your body will "ask" or will let you know in a way or another.

We must therefore adjust the diet based on the energetic and functional metabolism of the athlete, while having in sight that it must remain balanced.

In addition, liquid volume is to be adjusted before, during and after exercise to ensure proper hydration. An isotonic drink may be necessary during training because of its duration and intensity.

Here are some recommendations if you have intense workouts:
- ☞ If you have more intense workouts for a day, for a maximum of one hour per session, it is advisable to ingest a snack after each consisting of 1 g to 1.5 g of carbohydrates and 7 grams of protein per kg weight. This snack can be a briquette of milk and a banana for example.
- ☞ If you have intense sessions exceeding one hour, the snack is to be taken within 30 minutes after a workout if followed by another in the same day. This snack can be the one suggested above. Another snack is recommended after 2 hours, consisting of a slice of whole meal bread or cereal with soft cheese and unsweetened fruit juice or applesauce. The meal that follows is ideally time-framed from one to two hours after the precedent, and can be one of those recommended above.

In any case, if you are a sportsperson aiming performance, it is recommended that you consult a sports nutritionist to design a diet and hydration plan according to you and adapted to your height, weight, gender and discipline practiced.

Recommended diet for power / strength athletes

A strength sport is a physical activity that is based mainly on the strength of the individual. If this kind of sport has a long tradition all over the world, as in the Basque country, Scotland, New Zealand, Canada, through the "village Contests", the fact remains that Olympic events were born of these traditional sports. We find such and / or power contests in athletics: shot put, hammer and javelin, but also weightlifting or sumo.

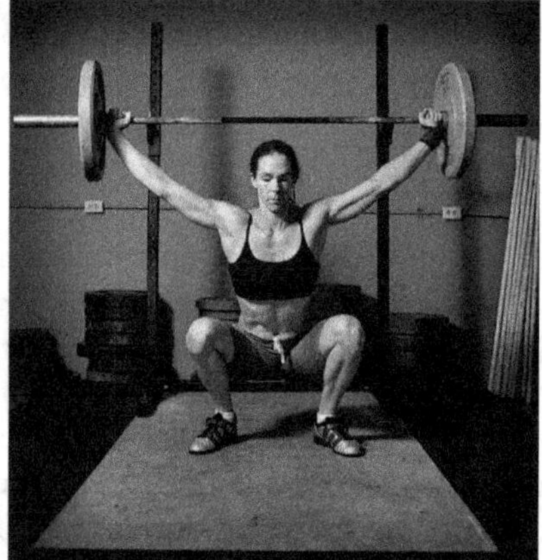

Basic nutrition principles for power sports / force sports

To gain strength and power, it is important to develop muscles, but not mainly in quantity rather in better quality. Indeed, not muscle mass is truly important in increasing strength, but the tone and quality of muscle fibers. In this quest, food plays an equally vital role and a sports nutritionist will advise you on the diet to follow.

Of course, each athlete must customize its "food program weight" according to the discipline s/he practices and progress goals in terms of performance. To gain strength, the sportsperson often will have to take muscle mass, but will carefully monitor his/her weight and fat percentage since the idea is to gain muscle without gaining fat. Progress tracking made a professional will help quantify muscle taking and quality (density, percentage of fat and muscle, etc.).

Nutrition before - during - and after exercise for the endurance athlete

It is important to never practice a sport fasting (without eating any food), because the benefit of weight training for example is directly proportional to the carbohydrate reserves of the muscles that will work during training. This is why one must adapt its nutrition depending on the day of training, but also the intensity of the session. In any case, here are some rules that may apply in order to give you an idea of the needs in terms of nutrition for a workout for strength / power:

☞ **Have a meal 4 hours maximum before the sport session**, composed of complex carbohydrates such as pasta or brown rice, or a cornmeal-based porridge like polenta. Adding a tablespoon of olive oil or nuts over pasta or rice will even more 'slow down' absorption of carbohydrates and improve its optimization during the session. The meal should also contain a source of (preferably animal) protein such as lean meat poultry (without the skin) or calf or white fish or an omelet of three eggs. A small applesauce or plain yogurt 0% after a meal. Finally you must drink a preferably alkaline water containing sodium to offset losses of minerals during the session via sweat.

☞ If the last meal was taken over 2:30 before training, it is advisable to consume **a snack from 1h30 to 2 hours before the session**. This snack should not contain fat. It may consist of a cup of oatmeal with some dried cranberries or raisins or dates or unsweetened pears and small fruit compote. A mineral-rich herbal tea can also be useful, hot or cold depending on the preference of the sportsperson.

☞ **Hydrate 30 minutes before the session** and during the session with plain water that can be enriched with a little fructose and some salt if it already does not naturally contains some in its formula (no more than 2 pinches salt / liter).

☞ During the session, **raw beet juice** can also provide more nitrates to the athlete by promoting dilation of blood vessels, allowing better blood supply to the muscles during exercise.

☞ After the session a **snack of 30 g of rice** (uncooked weight) cooked with 3 tablespoons of raisins or dried cranberries will stimulate insulin for muscle repair and rebuilding of muscle glycogen. Hydration continues to remain important because it is also involved in muscle repair.

Sample diet for a force / power athlete:

Here is an example of diet during the days of strength training for a 70 kg man who has a strength training program of 2 hours in the morning.

Breakfast

Food	kcal	carbohydrate g	protein g	fat g
total:	781			
1 cup skim milk, 0%	86	11	8.3	0.4
50g rolled oats	184	30	7	3
5 g dried cranberries	15	4	0.05	0.07
rice cake	150	26	3.9	3.5
1 hard-boiled Egg	78	0.5	6.2	5.3
2 slices whole wheat bread	140	30	11	1
1 banana	72	15.2	0.98	0.25
natural yoghurt, 0%	56	7.6	5.5	0.1

Morning snack: 1 fruit if more than 4 hours between breakfast and training.

During the session
It is advisable to hydrate properly. You can drink 150 ml isotonic drink every 15 minutes. Beet juice is also a good drink during the session.

After the session
After the session and during the following two hours it is advisable to have a snack - fruit juice, dried fruit, banana, yogurt, rice cake.

Food	kcal	carbohydrate g	protein g	fat g
total:	903			
1 avocado	322	17	4	29.4
150 g turkey breast	150	6	25.5	2
200 g whole-wheat pasta	246	52	10.5	1
50 g lettuce 1 case with walnut oil	8 90	1.63	0.5	0.08 10
baked beans	31	7.1	1.8	0.12
natural yoghurt, 0%	56	7.6	5.5	0.1

Afternoon snack: Fresh fruit (apple, orange, kiwi), dried (cranberries, goji or raisins) and / or nuts (walnuts, hazelnuts, almonds) + 1 dairy (yogurt drink milk or briquette).

Dinner

Food	kcal	carbohydrate g	protein g	fat g
total:	328			
100 g beet salad	61	9.6	1.6	2.2
1 portion of polenta (150g)	130	27	3	0.5
1 natural tuna portion	164	0	35.8	2.2
cottage cheese	103	2.68	12.5	4.5

You can add green vegetables if necessary.

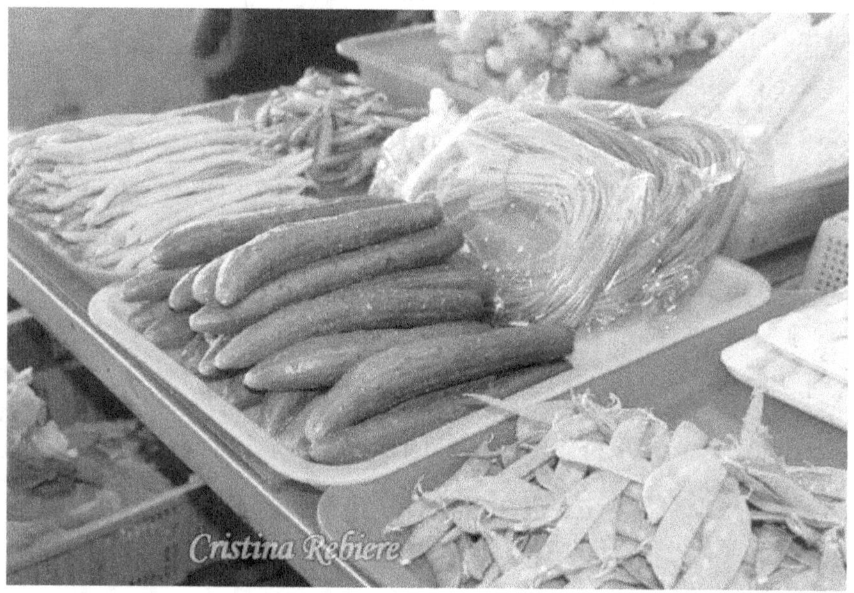

It is important to keep drinking until bedtime, as well as herbal teas. This will allow more effective muscle reconstruction. Finally, the quality of sleep is also important for a good recovery.

On days without training, we must favor a healthy, varied and balanced nutrition, with lots of fruits and vegetables, lean meat and fish, dairy products and whole grains.

Recommended diet for speed athletes

The "explosion" or explosive muscular strength is the ability of a muscle to trigger a maximal contraction in a very short time. This physical quality is to be found among the sprinters, weight or javelin throwers, boxers, weightlifters, etc.

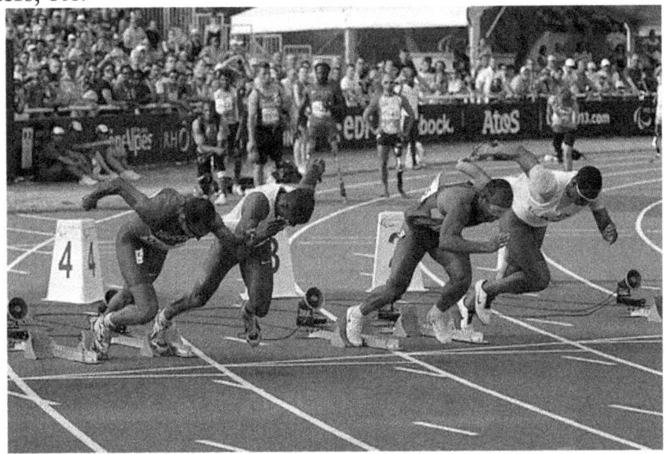

Basic principles of sports nutrition for speed / explosiveness sportspersons

Here are some principles to be adopted in the diet of an athlete in speed / explosiveness disciplines:

☞ Having a diet rich in energy intake up to 1.7 g of **protein** per kg of body weight per day, in order to support energy levels required by the maintenance of muscle mass. Protein is found primarily in **meat, fish and eggs, dairy products**, but also **legumes** and **whole grains**.

☞ Consuming adequate amounts of protein, but without excess.

☞ Consuming an adequate amount of **carbohydrates** to withstand the resistance workouts that use glycogen.

☞ Consume protein of a high quality source, between 20 and 25 g immediately after resistance training.

☞ Ensure the proper distribution of **protein intake** throughout the day.

☞ Carbohydrate intakes can be increased **4 to 5 days before the competition** in order to increase the amount of glycogen. In this context, it is important to consume **low glycemic index foods** at each meal, such as **whole grains** and legumes. It is also important to maintain blood sugar levels stable during the waiting phase, just before the test.

☞ During the **recovery** phase you need a fluid intake associated with a protein and carbohydrate food such as water with a cake or a recovery drink.

☞ Select foods that contain **protein with little fat** to avoid high consumption of saturated fat.

☞ Avoid erratic eating behaviors such as excessive weight loss before weightlifting competitions. Such behavior may disrupt the metabolism of the athletes and even cause health problems. Prefer a rational program well distributed in time if you want to change the category. However be aware that small weight losses in previous days the competition can be performed safely by following the advice of a nutritionist.

☞ For throwers or sprinters, choose a menu before the competition that makes you feel at ease during the trials.

The speed athlete's diet should allow an increase of the muscular strength but also and especially to "fill up" with the requested carbohydrates needs which will be transformed into energy during intense effort.

Finally, if you are unable to achieve the nutritional goals that you have set, it is better to seek advice from a sports nutritionist. It will bring you expert advice for the use of food supplements.

Sample diet for a speed / explosiveness athlete

Here is a sample diet before, during and after the competition:

Daily menu 5 days before the competition:

During the preparation of the competition a balanced diet should be favored, creating **glycogen reserves**, needed for the competition. It should bring about 400 grams of carbohydrates per day and 3000 kcal.

Breakfast:

Food	kcal	carbohydrate g	protein g	fat g
total:	779			
100 g cooked beets	43	7.2	2.3	0
100 g cooked mussels	150	4.4	13.8	8.25
100 g boiled brown rice	130	28	2.5	0.8
100 g lettuce 1 case with extra virgin olive oil	16 119	3.2	1	0.16 13.5
100g cooked green beans	77	9.9	2.37	4
1 portion of Camembert	114	0.17	7.5	9.2

Lunch:

Food	kcal	carbohydrate g	protein g	fat g
total:	779			
100 g cooked beets	43	7.2	2.3	0
100 g cooked mussels	150	4.4	13.8	8.25
100 g boiled brown rice	130	28	2.5	0.8
100 g lettuce 1 case with extra virgin olive oil	16 119	3.2	1	0.16 13.5
100g cooked green beans	77	9.9	2.37	4
1 portion of Camembert	114	0.17	7.5	9.2

Dinner:

Food	kcal	carbohydrate g	protein g	fat g
total:	418			
1 vegetable soup bowl	146	5.3	2.1	10.9
1 portion of polenta (150g)	130	27	3	0.5
50 g cream semi thick 4%	39	3.2	1.55	2.1
cottage cheese	103	2.68	12.5	4.5

Before a speed test:

We must ensure the stability of blood glucose, a good digestive comfort and good hydration.

It is advisable to have a snack 3 hours before the race, composed of:
- ☑ Juice
- ☑ yogurt
- ☑ cornflakes or oatmeal
- ☑ grain/cereal crispbreads

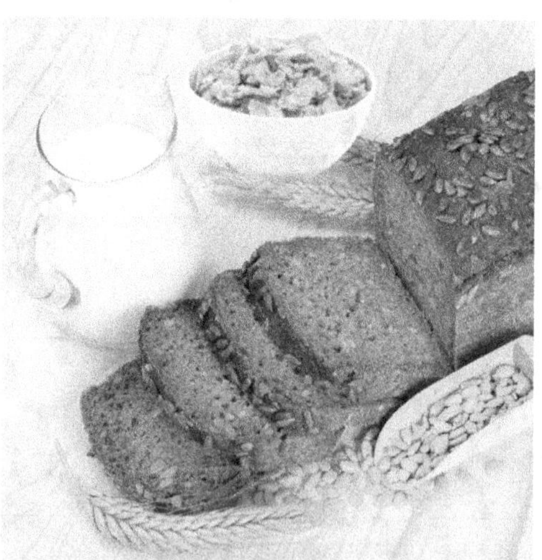

Until the warm up, you can drink isotonic drinks on a regular basis to ensure proper energy intake required for the test.

After the sport trial:

Energy reactions occurring in the muscles during the race does not stop instantly, so energy expenditure remains high after several hours. These reactions are burning additional sugars to be replaced **quickly** after exercise. Otherwise, the activity of the immune system, the rehydration of cells, kidney elimination work and repairing of muscle fibers are penalized.

One should also reduce as quickly as possible the acidity of the body. It is recommended to drink **beverages with high bicarbonates content**. Moreover, during the first 6 hours after the race, glycogen is reformed as quickly and easily. The intake of carbohydrates in liquid form is better tolerated by the intestines, so you should opt for hypotonic preparations: in addition to water mentioned above, you can drink diluted fruit juice or warm herbal tea honey. These drinks can be consumed during the first 30 minutes after exercise to allow time for the gut to regain its effectiveness. Then you can also eat solid contributions as dried fruit, whole meal bread or cereal, gingerbread or cookies.

If you want to know the properties of plants and herbal teas have ideas that you may find useful, you can take our little book **"90+ herbal teas to be in good health"** you can find on our website (https://OlivierRebiere.com) or on digital platforms.

Meals after exercise

The meal after sport exercise should be rich in carbohydrates to promote the establishment of an alkaline state, more suitable for a good recovery.

So you can make a meal of green vegetables (broccoli, green beans, etc.) or pulses (lentils,

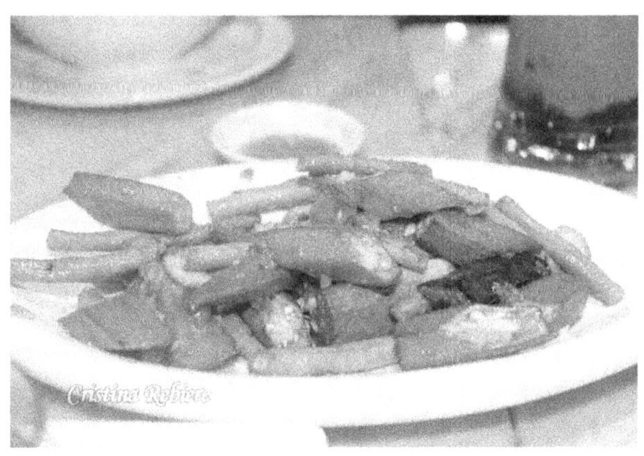

chickpeas), rice or pasta integrals, fruit (apple), a dairy product, an egg.

If it comes to dinner, you should avoid the consumption of meat or fish and drink a glass of milk or honey tea at bedtime to accelerate falling sleep and allow a restful sleep.

Effects of dietary supplements for athletes

Dietary supplements are foods whose purpose is to provide additional nutrients or vitamins, minerals, fatty acids or amino acids which are missing or are insufficiently provided by the normal diet of a person. They are supervised at European level by a 2002 directive, transposed into French law in the consumer code by a 2006 decree.

Dietary supplements are considered as "food" and are often subject to self-medication because they are not drugs. In addition, according to several studies, the French – for example – are quite fond of them as shown throughout the Inca 2 study (see the detailed article here https://www.anses.fr/fr/content/consommation-de-compl%C3%A9ments-alimentaires) which was conducted nationwide by the ANSES between 2005 and 2007. It found that 23% of adults and 12% of children consume food supplements all year or almost... These are fairly alarming proportions, knowing that few studies have been conducted on their actual effects on the human body.

You can find dietary supplements that have undergone extensive clinical studies and whose interest has been shown in the French Vidal dictionary of health professionals.

Effects and roles of dietary supplements

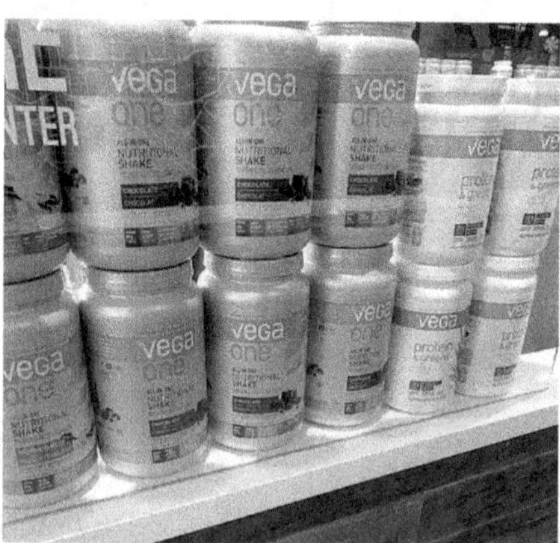

Photo: food supplements

Foods derived from modern agriculture are sadly depleted in nutrients and contain residues of pesticides or synthetic fertilizers, which significantly increase oxidative stress within our cells.

Food supplements, either in the form of capsules, tablets, capsules, ampoules or drinkable phials prevent some deficiencies or meet specific needs such as intensive or regular exercise. Similarly, the enrichment of certain foods can also fill this kind of deficiencies such as iron- or vitamin- fortified cereals or butters and margarines fortified with omega 3. The iodine-enriched salt is even more current and allows preventing cretinism and goiter.

However, a balanced and well-followed diet helps provide the nutrients needed for a normal person. Even in the case of athletes, a good knowledge of nutritional values and components that can harm in order to avoid them are able to ensure good coverage of their specific needs.

Some athletes rely on nutritional supplements to enjoy benefits such as:

➢ increase energy reserves;
➢ promote adaptation to training;
➢ allow for a more intensive preparation;
➢ improve performance during the competition;
➢ help recovery between training sessions;
➢ maintain good health and reduce interruptions to training due to chronic fatigue, injury or disease;
➢ provide an easy source of nutrients to consume when every day dishes are unavailable or difficult to consume.

Best known dietary supplements

Athletes have special needs especially depending on the discipline practiced, intensity, frequency and duration of training pushing the body beyond habitual consumption in both energy intake of nutrients and efforts and recovery.

Specific foods for athletes are usually developed to provide a convenient way to meet special dietary needs, helping them indirectly.
Some dietary supplements can be helpful, such as:

☞ **sports drinks** that allow adequate hydration while providing electrolytes and carbohydrates during training
☞ liquid foods rich in carbohydrates, protein, vitamins and minerals for a meal before the competition, for recovery after workouts or for a high-energy diet
☞ rich carbohydrates sports gels that are particularly useful during training
☞ "sports bars" (edible) that are the solid equivalent of liquid foods mentioned above.

The use of dietary supplements in pills, powders, light bulbs, etc. is quite common among athletes, but be aware that **very few of these products are** based on solid research, and some may even harm. This is why they should **carefully consider the risks and benefits of specific supplements before using them.**

However, some athletes may have a demonstrated deficiency in a certain vitamin or mineral essential, and when nutrition cannot fill it, a dietary supplement may be beneficial. For example, athletes with a diagnosed iron deficiency can take iron supplements, but only if a blood test shows that this extra supply is needed.

Protein bars

A quick source of energy can also be obtained from the consumption of **protein bars.** "**Sports bars**" have many qualities. Most bars for athletes are enriched with vitamins and minerals, or other ergogenic substances (for example carnitine and glutamine) and nutrient profiles tailored to specific needs - some are rich in protein, and are designed especially athletes who do strength training, others have a large amount of carbohydrates and are designed for endurance sports.

The choice of the bar type should be done **according to the type of training** you do. If you are an endurance athlete (marathoner, triathlete), higher grade bar in carbohydrates are recommended. However, these athletes can also benefit from the qualities of a bar rich in proteins, especially after a workout or a demanding competition where the body needs more protein intake to replenish the muscle structure. Similarly, strength or combat sports athletes can consume bars which are rich in carbohydrates before training for increased energy intake, but protein bars are most useful and commonly used to increase the protein intake that ensures the maintenance or development of muscle mass.

It is best to choose whole grains bars, which also contain seeds or nuts, or fruit pieces. These carbohydrate sources provide in most cases more than 3 grams of fiber per bar. These fibers are an important component for a healthy diet because they reduce the sugar absorption rate, provide satiety, maintain an environment conducive to the development of commensal flora and contribute to good intestinal transit.

A **well-chosen food** diet is more appropriate and will allow an adequate intake of vitamins, minerals and essential fatty acids.

Some supplements offer the prospect of improved performance for some athletes in specific competitions.

Creatine

It seems that creatine supplementation can increase the amount of high-energy phospho-creatine stored in muscle and enhance performance in sprints, but also could cause an increase in strength and / or muscle mass, useful in some sports. However, be aware that exceeding the recommended dose is not helpful as with all dietary supplements.

According to the **French Olympic Committee**[1] the ergogenic effects (producing energy and improving muscle performance) are real during very short exercises because they are associated with increased muscle creation in phosphorylated (phospho-creatine). However, the effects of creatine on performance for longer drives are much less convincing, even zero. The effect is zero also on muscle mass.

Creatine is normally found in **meat** and **fish**, but the effective doses of 10 to 20 g per day for 4-5 days for the loading creatine and 2 to 3 g per day to maintain, are difficult to recover by normal diet. This is why many athletes rely on creatine supplementation especially if they are vegetarians. It does not seem to be harmful to health. However, prolonged use or large quantities will cause extra work for the kidneys and therefore can eventually cause kidney disease. Creatine also generates weight gain that can affect the body. This overload may affect tendons, muscles and joints while causing injuries.

Creatine can be found in different forms: capsules, micro-granules or powder. It is also mixed with a protein called "whey".

The **French Society of Sports Nutrition** (in French: SFNS) and AFSSA agreed on the draft European directive that aims to not advise the use of creatine by athletes, because of allegations that do not seem to respect the sports ethics. See here https://www.nutritiondusport.fr/wp-content/uploads/2009/06/complements-alimentaires-chez-le-sportif-sfns-juin-2009.pdf

Magnesium

There are many dietary supplements containing magnesium. However, much of these products are pure marketing tools because there is no convincing method of accurate measurement of the amount of magnesium in the body. Therefore, it is rather difficult, if not impossible, to estimate magnesium intake additional benefits.

Magnesium reduces neuronal excitability and is involved in neuromuscular transmission, as well as in many enzymatic reactions.

The magnesium requirements are much higher in athletes than in normal people, about 350 mg for men and 300 mg for women (per day). With intensive training needs can be up to 550 mg / day. This high intake prevents the appearance of muscle cramps during intense efforts. Here are some **magnesium rich foods** (Magnesium content per serving of 100 g):

☑ Seafood - 410 mg

1 http://franceolympique.com/files/File/actions/sante/colloques/15eme/Andre XavierBIGARD.pdf

- ☑ sardines in olive oil - 467 mg
- ☑ cocoa - 150 to 400 mg depending on the concentration
- ☑ almonds - 250 mg
- ☑ Cumin seed - 366 mg
- ☑ sunflower seed - 364 mg
- ☑ sesame seeds - 324 mg
- ☑ whole meal bread - 80 mg
- ☑ brazil nuts - 370 mg
- ☑ roasted and salted peanuts - 168 mg

Caffeine

A small amount of caffeine in the range of 1 to 3 mg per kilogram of weight can help improve performance in prolonged workouts. It can also be useful in shorter workouts.

These doses can be covered by the daily amounts of coffee, green or black tea, other beverages or sports gels containing it. If you want to see a comparison of the caffeine content, you will find one here:
 http://www.thevert.com/cafeine/comparaison-the-cafe-coca/.
For example **a cup of coffee** provides **100 mg of caffeine**.
Higher doses of caffeine do not seem to further improve performance and may even have negative results such as gastrointestinal discomfort, a state of anxiety and / or excitement. As you know, high doses of caffeine can disturb sleep and thus prevent sufficient recovery.
Caffeine is present in combination with p-synephrine in food supplements marketed for sports performance and weight loss.

Omega 3

Several studies have demonstrated the positive effects of a diet rich in omega-3, which improves overall health and in particular that of the cardiovascular system. Omega-3s seem to preserve the joints, being in addition an excellent natural anti-inflammatory agent, which makes them very interesting for athletes, particularly in endurance and strength sports. The needs can be covered by the particular fish feed, fish livers and some oils. There are dietary supplements containing omega-3 fortified foods and even in this essential fatty acid such as margarines in particular.

Be aware that an overdose or a prolonged intake of Omega 3 can have adverse health effects, such as higher levels of bad LDL cholesterol, a decrease in immune and inflammatory responses in the body, a drop of blood glucose, especially in people with diabetes, etc.

Whey

Whey is a high quality milk protein that provides a rapidly digestible source of leucine and other essential amino acids.

A whey protein powder may be useful when repair and adaptation are the main needs for recovery or when a quick solution is needed to add quality protein to a sub-protein meal.

It seems that the proteins contained in whey have an important role in the reconstruction of muscle fibers that have undergone micro-tears during training. A 2010 article appeared on the occasion of a workshop organized by Nestlé speaks of the effectiveness of whey protein to stimulate muscle protein synthesis during recovery from exercise (see here https://www.karger.com/Article/Abstract/329287). However further studies have not been conducted to prove the effectiveness of these proteins.

Spirulina

Spirulina is a microscopic blue-green alga that grows in lakes and is rich in essential fatty acids, iron, calcium, magnesium and A, B and E vitamins. It is used as a dietary supplement while no clinical studies have confirmed its supposed properties. However the WHO seems to consider it as "the food of the future" and encouraged its production globally by considering it as a promising way to combat malnutrition.

Spirulina is very successful among athletes because it is supposed to help continue prolonged physical effort, increasing the resistance of the body including muscles, with its concentration of iron and protein. It seems to help reduce muscle cramps and the risk of injury resulting from the effort by delaying the production of lactic acid by the body. Its richness in iron and antioxidants promotes oxygenation of muscles, allowing better endurance by making cardio exercises most effective.

However, spirulina may have adverse effects especially in people prone to gout, kidney stones, or those with high blood levels of uric acid.

Finally, note that the price per kilo of spirulina is more expensive than foods that are equally interesting nutritionally, such as fresh and dried vegetables or vegetable oils.

If you want to know the opinion of the national food safety Food Agency, Environment and Labor (ANSES) on Spirulina, you can read the following article on their website:

(https://www.anses.fr/fr/system/files/NUT2014SA0096.pdf).

Ginseng, cayenne pepper, garlic, chamomile

All sportspersons are concerned with the prevention of overtraining, and seek to better adapt, resist stress, and recover faster. The **"adaptogens"** seem to meet these needs.

Ginseng and cayenne pepper in small doses, chamomile, garlic, are presented as having these beneficial effects and are even mentioned by the SFNS without their virtues being denied.

Antioxidants

The oxidative status of a given athlete varies depending on the discipline practiced, the intensity and level of training. It is more difficult to balance during intense exercise and while experiencing hypoxia. It is important to ensure that the mineral intake, vitamins and other nutrients brought by the daily diet remains consistent with the recommendations. The inputs of nutrients or antioxidants are evaluated by the physician or dietitian thanks to a food balance. Nutrients involved in the fight against free radicals are normally provided by a balanced and varied diet.

The NSF draws attention to supplementation that is not devoid of toxicity, especially during excessive inputs and unbalanced regarding one micronutrient that can interfere with the absorption or bioavailability of other micronutrients. Finally, another statement risk is that consumption of dietary supplements associated with a diet that already includes foods rich in vitamins and minerals may expose to overdoses.

Bicarbonate

In case of intense effort, the muscles produce lactic acid, bringing the energy to the athlete. But it is also the same substance that causes muscle pain and affects the functioning of the muscles. Sodium bicarbonate can neutralize excess stomach acidity, but also appear to counter the negative effects of lactic acid if it is taken in a dose of about 0.3 g per kg body weight before a competition. Bicarbonate supplements are widely used by athletes during intense workouts causing fatigue in minutes. We can find on a FIFA document on food supplements that "studies on simulations of typical activities of football players have proven the effectiveness of this product in certain cases." However, FIFA warns that the bicarbonate may cause gastrointestinal disorders (http://fr.fifa.com/mm/document/afdeveloping/medical/4.5.supplementsp2 2-24french_6388.pdf). Finally, it is also expressed on other dietary supplements that we already mentioned that there is no evidence or scientific studies proving their efficacy.

In all cases, the majority of food supplements are expensive and it is better to think carefully before eating consistently. You will need to analyze on your own if the benefits achieved through the consumption of this product actually give you an advantage in competitive sports without harming your health.

Scientific evidence of the dietary supplements effectiveness

Very few scientific studies have demonstrated the clinical efficacy of dietary supplements. Most of them are made on cell cultures or animals, but that does not really prove their beneficial effects on humans. It is the same thing for athletes.

The International Olympic Committee recommends necessary inputs for athletes through a balanced and well-chosen diet to meet their nutritional needs. It also recommends to athletes who might use dietary supplements to consider the effectiveness, cost, risk to health and performance, and the potential of a positive result for a doping test before considering their use.

A study made on 19 men and bodybuilders published in 2013 in the *Journal of the International Society of Sports Nutrition* (see here https://jissn.biomedcentral.com/articles/10.1186/1550-2783-10-36), concludes that the creatine supplementation during resistance training increases fat free mass and strength. It seems that creatine consumption immediately after training has superior effects for consumption before training regarding body composition and strength. Of course, the limited number of subjects participating in this study does not allow considering the results as scientific truths. A Dutch study that was conducted during the Olympic Games in Salt Lake City in 2002 was aimed at studying food supplements consumed by their qualified athletes. 69 food supplements were identified among those consumed by their delegation from which 14 contained non-specified stimulants on the respective product's labeling: 12 contained caffeine and 3, ephedrine. Another British study in 2015 on dietary supplements recommended for muscle-mass intake, found anabolic steroids in these products, without being notified on the labeling.

The European Union introduced rules to help ensure that dietary supplements are safe and appropriately labeled, as shown here (https://www.efsa.europa.eu/fr/topics/topic/food-supplements). They are regulated as foods and the legislation deals in particular with vitamins and minerals used as ingredients of food supplements.

The 2002/46/EC Directive establishes requirements for labeling and maximum and minimum doses of each vitamin or mineral added to supplements. However, it does not certify their effectiveness. It is important to note that the authorization of vitamin and mineral substances is done only after the assessment by EFSA (European Food Safety Authority) of a scientific dossier containing the necessary information about their safety and bioavailability. Therefore, these supplements are not dangerous to health taken in the indicated doses, but do not guarantee improved performance in the case of athletes. At most, these vitamins or minerals can fill the gaps that are induced by specific diseases.

Finally, the EFSA scientific group carried out the assessment of possible harmful health effects of micronutrient intakes at higher doses nutritional needs. They set the tolerable upper intake level (UIL) for various population groups. This represents the maximum daily dose taken over a prolonged period of a nutrient that is not likely to create a risk of adverse effects on human health.

The **French Society of Sports Nutrition** (in French: SFNS) advocates like other authorities regarding food for athletes, even those high-level, that a balanced and varied diet is recommended, especially in nutrient-dense foods to satisfy demonstrated specific needs. It did not recommend dietary supplements and believes that supplementation with products in attractive allegations on sports performance are not based on scientific or medical evidence. In addition it warns their use may pose a health risk for athletes and even for a positive doping test.

A study published in 2009 by the SFNS (Horde, "The use behaviors and dietary supplements in athletes") reveals that athletes are big consumers of food supplements for several reasons:

- ☞ biological impairment,
- ☞ clinical deficiencies,
- ☞ mismanagement of fat,
- ☞ energy intake deficiency of certain foods.

Expectations sports are therefore related to research performance and endurance.

The Research Institute of Wellbeing, Medicine and Sports Health (in French: IRBMS - https://www.irbms.com/les-complements-alimentaires) does not recommend dietary supplements for athletes. However some sportspersons, such as those following a vegan diet can benefit from iron supplements and B12-like vitamins if their diet does not cover nutritional needs related to efforts for training and competitions. On its website, the IRBMS draws attention to the difference between nutritional supplements and dietary supplements. The first are "dietary foods for special medical purposes" that aim to prevent or correct a state of malnutrition. They are available only in pharmacies with a prescription, and therefore their use should be done only under the supervision of a physician. Dietary supplements are not drugs and can be purchased without a prescription and are supposed to bring one or more substances that are missing or deficient in a normal diet.

A study was conducted in 2014 by the SFNS on safety of food supplements and the effort and recovery drinks. Only 7 effort drinks were secure among the 15 tested, and only 4 recovery drinks and on 9 evaluated.

Warnings against dietary supplements

Dietary supplements have few cons-indications in theory, because if they were authorized by EFSA to be marketed within the European Union, they are assumed to not present a danger to health. However, one has to consider allergies to certain plants of a few individuals and therefore athletes tempted to use them.

You should also consider the possible interactions between plants or components present in food supplements and the athlete's treatments prescribed by his/her doctor. It is best to talk with your doctor if you want to take supplements, especially if you are undergoing treatment to ensure the absence of interaction between the two.

FYI, vitamin E decreases the absorption of some drugs. Concentrated supplements of vitamin A are cons-indicated for patients with a history of cancer.

Products made of dehydroepiandrosterone (DHEA), soy, red clover, wild yam, flaxseed oil, chaste tree are cons-indicated in cases of gynecological, breast, and prostate cancers.

The **French Ministry of Health** presents some complementary food on its website, but is content to do it in a rather informative way and without really giving its opinion on the matter. However, it warns that "food supplements on the market are not subject to systematic prior scientific evaluation to ensure their quality." Authorities prefer to delegate this responsibility to distributors who must comply with standards... (see here http://solidarites-sante.gouv.fr/sante-et-environnement/denrees-alimentaires/article/complements-alimentaires)

Nevertheless, you are also cautioned on overdose due to exceeding the doses but also to concomitant taking of several supplements that may have ingredients in common.

The American **Food and Drug Administration** (FDA) presents on its website a more consistent advice as shown here: (https://www.fda.gov/Food/DietarySupplements/UsingDietarySupplements /ucm109760.htm). It is also recommends to avoid the combination of supplements among themselves or with drugs, but it also warns of risks to the operations and risks of overdose of A, D vitamins, or iron.

The French Ministry of Sports provides a brochure on food supplements, although this document is mad to the attention of pharmacists and not sportspersons who are the first concerned by these recommendations. It includes a warning on the fact that certain dietary supplements may contain dopant molecules and thus the existing risk for athletes who consume them, to be declared positive during a doping control. The substances mentioned are octopamine of Citrus aurantium and methylhexaneamine, "allegedly contained in extracts of Pelargonium graveolens (geranium)" which can make positive a doping control. We find the same recommendations for balanced and varied diet to meet the specific nutritional needs of athletes.

On the website of the French Order of Pharmacists, there is an insert for sportspersons (http://www.cespharm.fr/fr/Prevention-sante/Catalogue/Complements-alimentaires-Evitez-le-risque-de-dopageaccidentel-affiche) where the pharmacist must warn about possible contamination of food supplements by harmful substances.

A full article on the situation of food supplements is to be found on the Cairn.info website: https://www.cairn.info/revue-questions-de-communication-2015-1-page-79.htm#pa6.

The French Rugby Federation's Medical Committee manages the use of dietary supplements on the occasion of presenting nutritional support for athletes as part of their training. Nutritional support is based on nutritional protocols developed with the experts of the Federation and a selection of food supplements used during training was made based on profiles of players and workouts.

Confusion between isotonic drinks and energy drinks and adverse side effects

An **isotonic drink** meets the nutritional needs for the effort, being made of water, minerals, including sodium, and sometimes carbohydrates. It is adapted to long-term efforts.

By contrast, **energy drinks** bring other substances with potential effects on the body during a sports practice that leads to misuse and confusion about the carbohydrate content. If the carbohydrate content of an energy drink is between 20 and 80 grams of sugar per liter, in energy drinks quantities are much greater: between 100 and 120 grams per liter. Dr. Frederic MATON, President of the French Society of Sports Nutrition (SFNS) warns about this confusion. He explains that this excessive content is based on no nutritional justification whatsoever and increases the osmolarity of drinks, thus affecting the proper hydration of the sportsman. Energy drinks do not contain minerals, and do not compensate sweat losses during training or competition workouts or during the competition. They contain lots of B vitamins, but overdosing is useless. In the same document (http://franceolympique.com/files/File/actions/sante/colloques/16eme/Boi ssons_energetiques_ou_energisates.pdf), he says that these energy drinks are very acidic, with a pH between 3 and 4 which can result in digestive disorders, including stress. It also warns about the undesirable effects of caffeine such as tachycardia, hypertension, addiction, anxiety behavior and irritability. These side effects do not allow creating a favorable context athletic performance. Finally, Dr. Maton warns athletes on the risk factors induced by the consumption of energy drinks: dehydration, digestive disorders, heart disorders and maladjustment to the effort. The confusion between these drinks causes also kidney risk for athletes because of their diuretic effect. The water loss is accompanied by mineral loss, especially potassium and calcium.

Acknowledgments

We thank Wikipedia and Wikimedia websites for the resources used in the preparation of this work. We are grateful to all contributors without whom we could not have completed some of our articles. The "Watercolor Runner" image used within the SportPRO logo is provided by the Freepik.com website. And thank you to all the kind souls who offer online tools and free resources for use for those who still want to learn and improve!

Photo credits:

Photo 1.1: By Thorwald at English Wikipedia [Public domain], via Wikimedia Commons (Transferred from en.wikipedia to Commons.)

Photo 1.2: By Moyan Brenn from Anzio, Italy - Diet

Photo 1.3: By 821,292 [CC0 CC0 gold], via Wikimedia Commons

Photo 1.4: From BMI_fr.svg: Superwikifanderivative work: Sankarip (talk)

Photo 1.5: By Peggy Greb; edited by Fir0002

Photo 1.6: By Peter Mooney - London 2012: The Mens Olympic Marathon

Photo 1.7: By imagesbywestfall (imagesbywestfall), via Wikimedia Commons

Photo 1.8: By Clement Oral Lechat, from Wikimedia Commons

Photo 1.9: By Daylen - Own work, CC BY 4.0

Photo: By JKrabbe Wikipedia English - Transferred from en.wikipedia to Commons by using Naudefj CommonsHelper, Public domain.

Photo: By Haltero70 - Own work, CC BY-SA 4.0

Photo: By McSmit - Own work, Public domain

Authors

Cristina & Olivier Rebière first met at the age of seventeen in 1990 in Romania, shortly after the fall of the Berlin Wall and the Romanian Revolution of December 1989. They were married in 1993. Since then, these life adventurers had an existence full of surprises, with many professional experiences in several areas. Curious by nature and always ready to learn, they are interested in various topics, love traveling, entrepreneurship and writing. Their books are useful, practical, and addressed to the general public. Self-taught, they conducted extensive research in order to control the areas in which they exercised. They also developed numerous training sessions for both tree-climbing instructors, as for the construction of ropes courses and all aspects of operating such a business. In addition, Cristina is passionate about nature and interested for a long time to plants and animals as well as alternative medicines. In addition to the Nature collection which addresses a large audience, she designed training modules in naturopathy and has written numerous articles about healthy habits and wellness. In addition to this book, discover all Cristina & Olivier works on their website: http://www.OlivierRebiere.com!

Cristina Botezatu is a senior scientist specialized in neuromuscular aspects and preparation of the body for performance. Born and raised in Romania, where she coordinated scientific research and actively participated in the preparation of national teams for the Olympic Games in several sports, she holds a PhD in physical education and sport since 2014. Fascinated since childhood by the harmonious development of mind and body, she hosted many recreational and sporting activities for young people in our adventure park. At the National Research Institute for Sport in Romania, she devotes her energy and creativity to design new processes and motion analysis strategies to improve athletic performance.

She decided to work with us within this SportPRO collection to share her specialized experience in sports performance, the results of her work on biometrics research, neuromuscular control, nutrition, balance, strength and speed.

DIGITAL BOOKS

- Travel, Voyage Experience collection

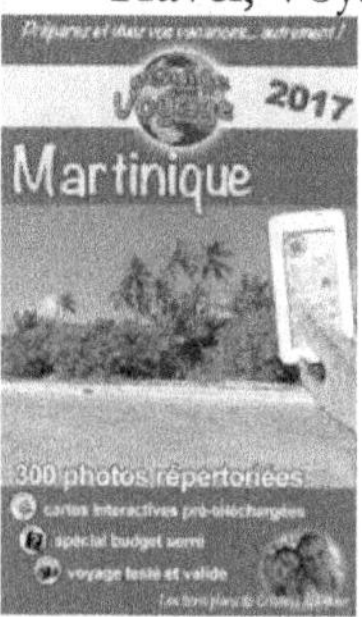

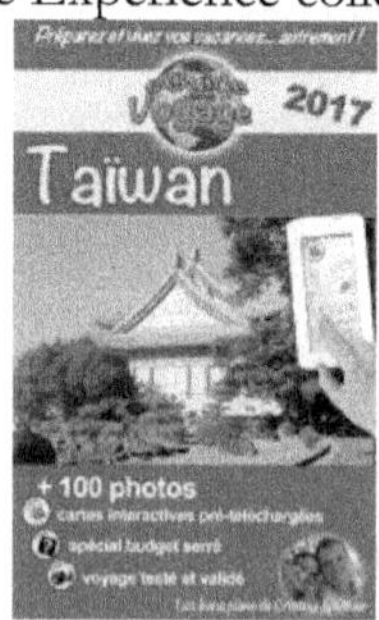

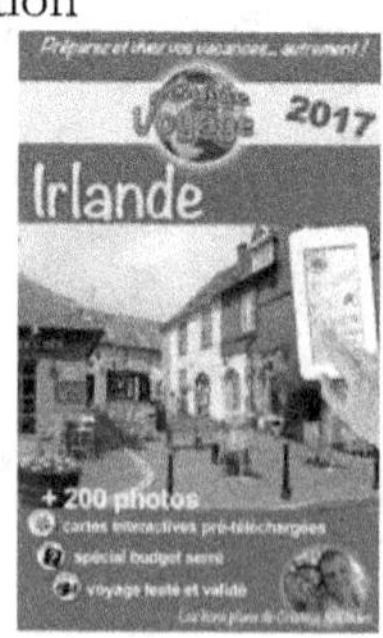

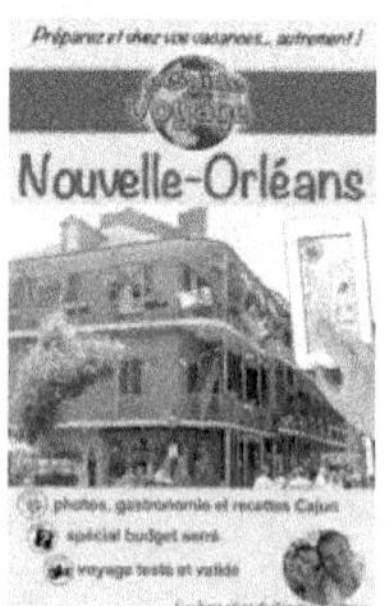

- Zen Attitude and Nature Passion collections

- Kids and Tools for Authors collections

- Team Building inside and Education collections